Vain Glorious

Vain Glorious

*A shameless guide for men
who want to look their best*

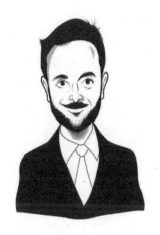

Jeremy Langmead
with Dr David Jack

———————————————

Published in the UK in 2021 by Short Books
an imprint of Octopus Publishing Group Ltd
Carmelite House, 50 Victoria Embankment
London, EC4Y 0DZ

www.octopusbooks.co.uk
www.shortbooks.co.uk

An Hachette UK Company
www.hachette.co.uk

10 9 8 7 6 5 4 3 2 1

Cover design © Andrew Smith
Cover Illustration © Antony Hare

Printed and bound in Great Britain by Clays Ltd, Elcograf S.p.A.

This FSC® label means that materials used for the
product have been responsibly sourced

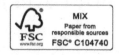

MIX
Paper from
responsible sources
FSC® C104740
FSC
www.fsc.org

"Vanity – definitely my favourite sin."

Al Pacino, *The Devil's Advocate*

Part One

by Jeremy Langmead

Part Two

by Dr David Jack

Part One

By Jeremy Langmead

Introduction

"SOMEDAY I WILL BE A BEAUTIFUL butterfly and everything will be better," announces Heimlich, the chubby German caterpillar, in *A Bug's Life*. This charming Pixar movie echoes sentiments not uncommon among humans, too. If only I had less fat, more money, a smaller nose, a bigger house, then everything would be okay, we tell ourselves. Sometimes this dissatisfaction with our lot drives us to success; at other times to utter despair.

Ultimately, most of us are aware that those outward signs of our internal struggles are not the key to change. A new nose (rhinoplasty is one of the top three cosmetic surgeries men request) is not going to transform your life but, perhaps, it will make you feel a little bit better about yourself. And if so, that's not necessarily a bad thing. As Dr Howard Murad, one of the world's leading skin and healthcare specialists, says: "If having fewer wrinkles or a little more hair is going

13

to make you feel better, then that can add to your health."

Until recently, male motivation for looking good or strong was often born from an inherent desire for us to feel and appear more successful, competitive, virile and powerful; what some now refer to as toxic masculinity. But that's changing. There's a new generation that wants to feel comfortable with who they are; internally and externally: that might mean a simple haircut, or some dermal filler to firm up a jawline or, for others, something more intrinsic, such as a change of gender identity. And, as a society, we've become less judgmental and more accepting of those that feel differently to us.

At a recent supper with my 27-year-old son, his girlfriend and some friends of ours, the subject of trans people, gender expression and the debate over bathrooms came up. My son can't even believe it's a subject being discussed; he's puzzled as to why people still care about the sexuality or gender of others. While informed debate is important, later that night I reflected on how we must welcome the fact that a generation has grown up to believe as he does. I can remember picking him and his brother up from a party in London – they must have been 10 and 13 years old at the time – when one of their school friends came out of the front door wearing a dress. "Why was Ben wearing a dress?" I asked Oscar, a bit bemused, during the drive home. "Oh he always likes wearing dresses when he's not at school," he shrugged. And that was that. Admittedly, that was in north London. It's not the same experience for everyone. But the loosening of the rules for how men can, and want to, behave and look is gaining more momentum than ever before.

At my goddaughter's 16th birthday party recently, two of the boys from her school were wearing foundation, eyeshadow and tinted lip balm. For them, wearing make-up wasn't about being gay, or non-binary; it was about emulating their favourite K-pop groups. The stars of those South Korean boy bands have no qualms about wearing make-up – they use it to hide blemishes, even out skin tones, and as a fashion statement. And their legions of fans across the world are happily following suit. Many young South Koreans find it puzzling that their counterparts in the West are still a little more reticent; especially when you think that back in the 1980s it was British pop stars such as Adam Ant, Boy George and Duran Duran who pioneered the look in the first place. In fact, the latter's keyboard player, Nick Rhodes, 58, still does.

But what about the rest of us? After all, our politicians have relied on a little dab or two in this area for some time (Emmanuel Macron reportedly spent £22,000 on make-up in his first three months of office; while Trump relied on an unidentified smudgy orange substance which one hopes costs considerably less). And in order to obey social distancing rules, middle-aged, male television presenters and newscasters had online tutorials to teach them to apply their own make-up before appearing in front of the cameras.

Esquire magazine recently published a piece about men's make-up, renaming the products and treatments as "guyliner", "menscara" or "menicures" to make them sound a little bit more palatable for some of its readers. Look around the high streets of the country's major cities and you'll notice how many men in their early twenties are choosing to wear make-up; hopping on and off buses and tubes without batting a fake eyelash. Equally visible are the lusty lads appearing on reality TV shows, comfortable being filmed indulging in ab-friendly gym sessions before applying tinted moisturisers, plucked-eyebrow gels and lashings of fake tan. And less visible, but on the increase, are the "regular guys" who just want to look a little bit better. For example, retailers such as John Lewis and Mr Porter stock a men's cosmetic brand called War Paint For Men, founded by a 34-year-old father of two, Danny Gray; its sales have exceeded expectations.

Internet shopping has helped the more cautious of us feel a tad braver – with both the clothes we buy and the grooming products we try. You can order and experiment with what you've bought in the privacy of your own home without feeling judged. War Paint's website features video tutorials with silver-haired sixty-somethings demonstrating how to apply under-eye concealer or anti-shine ointments. The men's personal-care market, as it's known in the business (understandably everyone's trying to avoid using the word "grooming" these days), has been predicted by Allied Market Research to be worth $166b by 2022. In China, male beauty and skincare is one of the country's fastest-growing consumer product segments. "Chinese men are more open to experimentation," said the AMR report.

Now that more of us see our puzzled faces appearing on video conferences, and are all too aware of what we look like today, perhaps we too will become a little braver with our beauty regimes. Although, of course, some will resist. The TV presenter and columnist Jeremy Clarkson wrote in his *Sunday Times* column that he had hoped the Covid-19 pandemic would have put an end to us all caring about our looks; months of lockdown, he argued, had made us all feel that we could do away with haircuts, treatments and cosmetics. He's particularly against men having hair transplants: "A hair transplant is not like a penis-enlargement operation. You can't hide it away in your trousers and only reveal it to people who've never seen it before. It's on your head. So, one minute you have see-through hair, and the next it's as though the Forestry Commission has been round. We are going to notice that, and when we do, we are going to laugh."

Clarkson's funny because he creates a scenario based on extremes, but he's wrong about the fact that if you get a hair transplant everyone will laugh at you. It's no longer a taboo subject. In the same week that Clarkson wrote that column, the comedian Jimmy Carr appeared on television sporting a new hairline. When the chat show host asked him about it, Carr replied that he had enough hair, it was just in the wrong place. "My hair was socially distancing from my forehead and I'd had enough of it," he added.

Surely it's what's on the inside that really counts though, you ask. And increasingly we are aware that, yes, it is: not just in spirit but in substance. We've been educated to believe that nutrition, exercise and mental wellbeing affect how we look as well as how we feel. And we've learned that the way we behave and treat others, and the paths we choose to take, have more consequences than perhaps ever before. But, does that really mean we can't play around with the outside, too? If who we are is the person inside, and our bodies are just the casing we come in, what's the harm in a teeny-tiny bit of embellishment? Who doesn't sometimes want to polish or place a couple of stickers on their suitcase? When we move into a new house – especially if it's a period one – we'll peer around and acknowledge that we mustn't meddle with the original ceiling mouldings and architraves, but we don't hesitate to discuss updating the walls with a new lick of paint or change of wallpaper.

Charles Baudelaire, the 19th-century French poet and essayist – I know, he's a bit of a student thesis filler, but he's on my side – wrote an essay called "In Praise of Artifice" in which he argued that: "Everything beautiful and noble is the result of reason and calculation. Crime, of which the human animal has learned the taste in his mother's womb, is natural by origin. Virtue, on the other hand, is artificial… Good is always the product of some art. All that I am saying about Nature as a bad counsellor in moral matters, and about Reason as true redeemer and reformer, can be applied to the realm of Beauty. I am thus led to regard external finery as one of the signs of the primitive nobility of the human soul." I think he makes a good point. And he wasn't a vain or flippant man. Look at his profile pictures…

Beauty may be skin deep, but how we feel about the way we look often dives so much deeper. And an interest in how one looks, or a play with gender fluidity, does not have to be at odds with what one thinks or achieves. Look at the genius of Eddie Izzard, or Grayson Perry and his female alter ego Claire. Or think back to the 17th century and Louis XIV's brother, the Duke of Orléans, known as Monsieur, who enjoyed the company of men, as well as that of his two wives, and would often turn up to balls in full female attire. And yet on the battlefield he was both courageous and skilled, leading the French army to numerous victories. The only criticism of his soldiering skills was that he was often a little late to battle since it took him rather a long time to get dressed.

In the same vein, so to speak, was the British couturier and dandy Bunny Roger. He fought bravely in Italy and north Africa in the Rifle Brigade during the Second World War, returning home commended for his courage in rescuing a fellow officer from a burning building. Roger was modest about his achievements and admitted that he'd sit in the trenches reading a copy of *Vogue* magazine until it was time to lead a charge on the enemy.

So don't let anyone make you change the way you look, but neither let them stop you changing aspects of yourself you don't like if you're sure it's safe and right for you. If clothes, cosmetics, beauty regimes or treatments make you happy, enjoy them.

In this great big bonkers world we find ourselves living in, with so much more beyond our control than ever before, does it matter if a man spends a long time looking in the mirror when he's washing his hands? Is it a crime to spend some of your funds on moving follicles from the back to the front of your head, where a map of Ireland has begun to emerge? Is it shameful to crave a dab of Botox to stop your forehead looking furious? Nobody bats an eyelid (that might be the Botox) if you take an ibuprofen pill to ease a headache, Imodium to calm a stomach, or an Instagram filter to get more Likes. So why can't we use lotions, potions and clothes to feel better, too?

Being insecure about the way you look, or just feeling it could be improved upon, is exhausting enough without being made to feel bad about it. Critics of those who fight the ageing process – actually "fight" is too harsh a word, let's say bicker with it – point out that we should accept that our faces and bodies change as we get older. And they're right. We do have to accept that. And in fact there are many reasons to embrace some of those changes and the positives they bring with them. But some of age's comrades are a little less welcome. Ear hair isn't especially pleasing. Eating a Toblerone and shortly afterwards seeing it poking out above your waistline is a tad frustrating. Your eyelids deciding to take it easy and casually hang over your eyeballs is uncalled for. And my nose didn't need to get any bigger, but, yep, there it grows.

It should not be frowned upon if we try to make that journey to decay a little more comfortable. If we have the desire and can be arsed, why shouldn't we get the train, rather than a plane, into old age? Hop aboard the Belmond Orient Express rather than Easyjet. Ease ourselves into looking older rather than bungee-jump into it.

Many men now see it as business critical to look fit for purpose for as long as possible. More of us live longer, more of us rejoin the dating scene later in life, more of us want our earning power to last well beyond our early sixties.

And even though we are now more open-minded, better educated and considered about the lifestyle choices we make – whether it's eating less meat, drinking fewer beers, ensuring we exercise regularly or slapping on a bit of moisturiser in the morning – there's still so much more we're not quite sure about. Just look at the shelves laden with vitamins and food supplements in your local pharmacy, the rise of the vitamin drip clinic, the plethora of non-surgical cosmetic procedures on offer on the high street, the in-depth analysis you now get from a BUPA check-up… it's made it all a little overwhelming. And, as with health, Google isn't always helpful when you search for beauty advice. Search the symptoms of man flu and you'll find you've probably got Covid or typhoid. Tap in how to get rid of eye bags and you'll see a picture of a man wearing more bandages than Lazarus.

The trick with all the potions, tweaks and treatments available today is to know what works best for you, and to know when to say no. If you get it right, you'll look like you've had a good night's sleep or a relaxing holiday; if you get it wrong someone will ask you what you've had done. Often it's just a good haircut, an eyebrow tidy and a nicely tailored jacket that will do the trick; sometimes it's a bit of cosmetic work on your teeth and a jab of Botox, and for those feeling braver there's the possibility of fat freezing to help slim the waistline or a syringe of dermal filler to give your face a bit of volume.

Since I was a teenager, I have paid more attention than is perhaps healthy to my appearance. I have even made a career out of keeping up appearances – launching the *Sunday Times Style* supplement, editing magazines like *Esquire* and *Wallpaper*, being one of the founders of the men's e-commerce business Mr Porter and writing a grooming column for *The Times*'s LUXX magazine. In that time I've learned that there are a lot of clinics and practitioners out there who will promise you all sorts of solutions that I'm afraid are too good to be true; and others who will recommend fixing elements of your face or body that are already picture perfect. You need to find someone you can trust and who champions a natural approach to aesthetic and anti-ageing treatments. A good rule is to only trust someone who has been personally recommended to you; someone whose own face doesn't look tampered with; someone whose other clients don't look like startled aliens. Dr David Jack is one of those doctors. A member of the Royal College of Surgeons of Edinburgh, David studied medicine, anatomy and embryology before working for the NHS for many years, where he trained in specialist posts including burns, microsurgery, internal medicine, hand surgery, surgical dermatology and skin cancer. He is now established as one of London's leading aesthetic doctors, operating from his own Harley Street clinic.

I first met David when interviewing him for a piece for *The Times* newspaper. His gentle manner, less-is-more approach to his craft and deep understanding of the physiology of the face put me at ease when I had my first Botox treatment with him. David is a firm believer that injectables should be used to replace volume that has been lost and only ever relax muscles, not to create anatomically unnatural structures or paralyse muscles in the face. His is a holistic approach: he is as interested in skin health (he has his own range of skincare products and supplements) as he is in cosmetic treatments. On occasion I have been to visit him at his clinic and he has sent me away again saying that nothing needed doing. A waste of a cab fare, but the sign of a good doctor.

In this book I will walk you through the insecurities, pressures and processes that shape how we men dress, look and see ourselves; plus offer some tips and tricks, for both inside and out, that will address the bits and bobs that tend to bother us. Dr David Jack, meanwhile, will act as your own private consultant. He will expertly explain what happens to your face and body as you age and the treatments you can realistically have that will take the edge off ageing without making you look "done". He will provide the answers to questions you may have felt uncomfortable about asking others.

What we are not going to do is tell you how to brush your hair, cut your nails, iron a shirt or apply a moisturiser, because we're going to assume you're not 12 years old. The easiest way to describe our approach, perhaps, is to compare it to how you feel when you walk into your kitchen the morning after a dinner party. You look at the mess in front of you, try and recall whether the evening was worth it or not, and then gingerly begin to tidy up.

Towards the end of *A Bug's Life*, Heimlich emerges from his chrysalis looking almost exactly the same. He has barely transformed into a butterfly at all. He's still a chubby caterpillar but with tiny wings that don't have a chance in hell of lifting him off the ground. But Heimlich is too excited to notice. "I'm finished. Finally I'm a beautiful butterfly!" he exclaims, flapping his useless wings. So that he doesn't notice their ineffectiveness, Heimlich's insect friends lift him off the ground so that he believes he's truly flying. "Auf Wiedersehen!" he shouts joyfully to everyone below.

If you have friends like Heimlich, lucky you. If you don't, read on.

Chapter 1

Face Ache

My first, unintentional, foray into the world of skin rejuvenation was at the age of 42. Despite living in London, my job required me to travel each month to New York for a few days. It sounds inconvenient, but I loved the city and had a few friends who lived there. One weekend I arrived in Manhattan, a little jet-lagged, and my friend Andrew peered at me over dinner and said that he'd book me an appointment with his dermo (what New Yorkers call dermatologists). What a treat, I thought, a revitalising facial would be just what I needed to kickstart the week.

The following morning I arrived at the clinic, which looked disarmingly spartan for a spa, and waited for my appointment. The dermatologist called me into his office, made some polite small talk and started peering very closely at my face. He asked me to smile, and then to frown. I was expecting a hot towel to be wrapped around my face at this point but, hey, this was New York. He then took a marker pen and drew some black points on my forehead. This was clearly going to be a very precise facial. And then he picked up a small syringe. It was at this point that he saw how alarmed I looked. "Have you had Botox before?" he asked.

A normal person at this point would have said that there had been a terrible misunderstanding, apologised for the inconvenience and hailed a cab. Not me. British and polite, and not wanting to waste anyone's time or money, I told him that I hadn't had Botox before but to please go ahead as I didn't want to hold him up any further.

Ouch ouch ouch. I felt it. Not lots, but there must have been about eight separate pricks with a tiny needle into my forehead and the space between my eyebrows. Mercifully, it was over quickly. The doctor then gave me some ice, wrapped in a thin cotton flannel, and told me to keep it pressed on my forehead for 10 minutes to help alleviate the swelling. It would, he said, take three to seven days for the Botox to start taking effect; and about two weeks before I saw the full effects. I tried not to look concerned, but then realised this might be one of the last times I could look sad for a few months and so decided to make the most of it.

I returned to the reception area where, while holding an ice pack to my punctured forehead, I sat down and pretended everything was normal. After a few minutes, I built up the courage to peer into the mirror on the wall behind me. I had eight little lumps on my forehead, like bee stings; a couple of them sporting tiny particles of dried blood. I couldn't head into the outside world looking like this and so sat back down and googled.

According to the American Board of Cosmetic Surgery, over seven million people in the US each year receive Botox injections. Why, you may wonder, do so many of us inject the botulinum toxin into our faces? At first glance, it sounds less than ideal: botulinum toxin-type A is one of the strongest poisons around. The clinical syndrome of botulism, which is often lethal, typically occurs following either a wound infection or eating undercooked or improperly stored food.

It was a Belgian microbiology professor, Emile Van Emerngem, who first identified the pathogen in 1895. A piece of cured ham had poisoned 34 people at a wedding, three of whom had died. He gave the toxin its name, *C botulinum*, from the Latin word for sausage (sausage poisoning was common in Germany at the time).

It took almost another century for it to become what we now know as Botox. And its journey to cosmetic nirvana was an accidental one, brought about by a number of different doctors harnessing the toxin's ability – in microscopic doses – to effectively block the signals from nerves to muscles. This prevents the targeted muscles from contracting, which can ease certain muscular conditions.

The San Francisco-based ophthalmologist, Alan Scott, for example, discovered it could be used to treat patients suffering from crossed eyes or double vision. And Jean and Alistair Carruthers, a married opthalmologist and dermatologist couple from Canada, chanced upon the fact that patients being treated for involuntary closure of the eyelids with injections between the eyes and in the upper halves of their faces, had less prominent frown lines post-treatment. They soon realised how this could be used for pure cosmetic enhancements, too.

Scott initially managed to source the toxin from Ed Schantz, a military biochemist who had worked for the US biological weapons programme and was then based at the University of Wisconsin. Taking into consideration that the botulinum toxin is on the US Centers for Disease Control and Prevention's list of heavily regulated substances that could "pose a severe threat to public, animal or plant health", we're lucky that Scott and Schantz were careful; especially as Schantz would send the crystallised toxin to Scott in a metal tube through the post.

In 1991, after reports about its cosmetic uses were published in various medical journals in the late 1980s, the pharmaceutical company Allergan bought the rights from Scott to develop Botox, then called Oculinum, for cosmetic and therapeutic treatment.

A year later, the US Food and Drug Administration (FDA) approved Botox Cosmetic, botulinum A toxin, to temporarily improve the appearance of moderate-to-severe glabellar (frown) lines. Botox was born.

Today, Botox is manufactured at a high-security plant in the small town of Westport, county Mayo, in Ireland. The "source drug" is kept at a secret location in the States and so the small amount of the purified toxin needed to make the world's supply of Botox for an entire year – the size of an aspirin – is flown to Ireland on a private plane, with bodyguards. Minuscule quantities of the drug are then combined with a saline solution and distilled into 80 million vials, which are then shipped around the world each year.

It's big business. When Allergan first bought Botox, they thought they could do $10m in sales a year; in 2020 they had actually grown to around $4b. In May 2020, Allergan was bought by AbbVie, a US biopharmaceutical company, for $63b. AbbVie's CEO justified the price by stating that: "It's highly unlikely that we would see a biosimilar against Botox for a long, long time, if ever." Although the competitors were already circling, with lower-cost and longer-lasting alternative toxins reportedly almost syringe-ready.

The length of time a Botox treatment lasts (usually three to four months) and the amount it costs (around $300/£250 per area at a top clinic) are the drawbacks. Wrinkle erasing doesn't come cheap. And if it does, to be honest, you should make sure you've seen the work on other people first. Whoever administers your Botox should be a medical practitioner and on a recognised register to show that they've met the correct standards in training, skills and insurance.

If not administered properly, there can be side effects. Botox injected into the wrong set of muscles, for example, can cause a temporary droopiness of the eyebrow or eyelids. This droopiness eventually corrects itself as the Botox dissipates, but for a few weeks can make you look as if you're half asleep, or as if you're winking at everyone (not ideal if you work in an office). And too much Botox will freeze all the muscles in your forehead and give you what's become known as "plastic face" – an inability to show any expression. Someone could propose marriage to you and you would still only be able to stare back at them blankly. After Hollywood and reality stars were derided for overindulging on Botox, most practitioners have now learned to hold back on the doses, even if clients ask for more.

There are exceptions, however. I spoke to one Botox practitioner who told me about a male client who asked him to inject enough Botox to ensure his face didn't move at all. As any good practitioner should, the doctor refused the request, saying it would look unnatural and he couldn't do that to anyone. The client insisted that this was what he wanted. Eventually, the doctor agreed to give a little more Botox than he thought advisable, but not as much as the man wanted, with the caveat that when the Botox had kicked in properly, he still wasn't happy he could come back for free. Two weeks later, the man returned for a top-up. Are you sure? implored the doctor, it looks fine as it is. It turned out that the patient was one of the country's leading poker players; a face unable to show any expression was key to him winning. His (immobile) face was his fortune.

Fifteen minutes after my first, unexpected, Botox treatment, the bee sting swellings had disappeared, I had wiped the specks of blood from my face, and caught the subway home. Everything seemed normal once more. But the fact remained that in a few days' time I would no longer have frown lines and I would no longer have a furrow of fury between my eyes. I would instead have a smoother forehead and a fresh-eyed expression. I didn't know whether to be happy or sad. I didn't know whether my face would be able to depict whichever of those two emotions I chose. I didn't know whether I would regret that I'd erased a part of my face's own history. I might have got one of those frown lines when I discovered that Take That had split up; the furrow between my eyes could have been the result of watching too many episodes of *Lost*. Both would soon be gone – memories erased by a toxin.

But the truth is many of us erase the bits of our lives we don't like all the time; sometimes physically, other times psychologically. Sitting on the subway in New York, I realised that I had been editing things out nearly all my life. But, I like to think, sparingly, and with caution. I have a Botox top-up twice a year and, so far, nothing has gone wrong. It's one of those easy, lunch-break tweaks; the cosmetic equivalent of a KitKat. No-one but me really notices when I've had it done. The injections I have, from someone I trust on London's Harley Street, are subtle. My forehead still moves, but less so; the crow's feet at each side of my eyes (my eye wrinkles are my "weak" point) are less pronounced; and the frown line is softer. If I do ever get a comment, it's usually someone asking if I've had time off, or lots of sleep. The Botox makes me look more rested. I like that. Especially as I'm not.

Naturally, some men of my acquaintance are unsure about

Botox. Not the aesthetics of it, necessarily, but the long-term effects of injecting a toxin into your face. They worry, understandably, that temporarily paralysing your facial muscles could eventually cause them to weaken and even collapse. There is no evidence that this can happen. And after a couple of decades of usage, you would expect to see some signs of this potentially being the case if it were true.

A study published in *Pharmacology*, an international journal that reviews the latest findings and concepts in drug development and therapy, ran a report on repeated injections of botulinum toxin for cosmetic use. It cited a retrospective study of 943 patients, each of whom had had at least three consecutive Botox injections for the treatment of lines on the upper face, and reported that there was no evidence of cumulative adverse effects. In one case, the journal noted, a patient who regularly received botulinum toxin-type A for frontal and glabellar lines for a period of 13 years had also had no adverse effects.

The only negative report I could find was a study published by the University of Zurich in which scientists measured electric signals inside the brain before and after a Botox treatment. If we wrinkle our foreheads or raise our eyebrows, we stimulate the brain via the many facial nerves. Therefore paralysing these muscles could, they argued, reduce brain reactions, including impulses coming from the hands. Allergan, unsurprisingly, responded that they hadn't noticed any loss of sensitivity in people's hand, after a Botox injection. The university's research continues.

Apart from that, there seems little else to not to be able to frown about.

Chapter 2

Of Beards and Bushes

THE LEAST EXPENSIVE, AND MOST EFFECTIVE, way to give yourself less to worry about when it comes to your skin is to carry on wearing a face mask after they're no longer considered mandatory. They have been a lifesaver in more than one way. With only your eyes peering out from over the mask, scarf or bandana, there's a lot less of you on show (although those of you who, like me, wear spectacles will have discovered that an unfortunate side effect of masks is that they tend to make your glass lenses cloud over; no-one can see you, yes, but neither can you see anyone or anything).

Before Covid masks, beards were the cheapest skincare solution for men. Forty per cent less face to worry about. A good beard – by which I mean the skin mass it covers rather than its furry depth – requires relatively little maintenance work if kept short (using, say, the number 5 setting on your trimmer). It's only when whiskers are allowed to wander –

like the hipster ones that started sprouting all over the face in 2007 – that you need to start messing with beard oils and specialist combs. These fuller beards tend to dry out the skin, catch bits of your lunch, get caught up in tie knots and irritate the people you kiss. Something in between stubble and full beard – a little more unkempt than Tom Ford, a little tamer than Jason Momoa – is probably the right balance to aim for.

Occasionally, it's helpful to visit a proper barbershop – ideally a Turkish one – to keep the shape of your beard in check. It's sometimes hard to judge the full shape of one's own beard from looking in the mirror (although a few stealth selfies from different angles can help with this), and so it's good to get a professional to give you some perspective. However, in my experience, the pro beard tamers tend to look upon beard shaping as an art, and you come away with something that looks a little too "designed". I think it's best to let your beard look as much as possible as if it grew in the shape that nature intended.

And if you have a weak chin, as I do (medical name: retrogenia) – which will only become more prominent as you age – a beard disguises the fact; when you hit your fifties and your jawline sags a little, a beard gives the impression otherwise; if your lips are a tad thin, let your beard creep over the border. It's the DIY facelift you can grow at home.

Years ago, when I was working for a British magazine called *Elle Decoration*, we were photographing the late romantic novelist, Dame Barbara Cartland, at her grand

and ornate home in Hertfordshire. Ms Cartland insisted on doing her make-up herself. I watched, in wonder, as before applying her famously pronounced facade, she and her assistant attached two strips of sticky tape to her cheeks. The sticky tape was used to pull up the skin on each cheek into her hairline to make her face appear tauter; over the sticky tape she then applied heavy foundation and powder. When we received the un-retouched photographs a few days later, you could still see the sticky tape shining through. We kindly airbrushed it out.

Facial hair has grown in and out of fashion over the last few decades. It was popular in the 1960s and 1970s as a hirsute act of rebellion against the previous generation's clean-cut conformity. Hippies, beatniks, yogis, musicians and students grew goatees, sideburns, moustaches, even neck beards. The trouble was that men were so excited to rediscover facial hair, and the myriad variations it could grow into, that they just watched it flourish on their faces without considering aesthetics or hygiene. It was out of control, like Japanese knotweed. I wonder if another reason for its untethered growth back then was purely practical: try having a contouring shave after smoking a big fat joint or dropping a tab of acid.

The end of the 1970s also saw the end of moustaches and beards. The success of the Village People – with its moustachioed band members (in particular Glenn Hughes with his resplendent horseshoe example); the bearded man in a sexual embrace on the cover of Alex Comfort's bestselling 1972 manual, *The Joy of Sex* (it went on to sell over 12 million copies), and the fact that the gay community, following the Stonewall riots of 1969 in particular, adopted the moustache as a sign of masculinity and strength, all led to its demise as an act of alternative rebellion. Then the 1980s, with its clean-cut Wall Street ambition and the onset of the HIV crisis, came along. It was the final straw.

Like every fashion since the 1970s, we've seen beards bounce in and out of style every few years. They re-emerged as scruffy tufts, much like Shaggy's in *Scooby-Doo*, in the 1990s, with the grunge movement; again in the 2000s with the hipsters' love of lumberjacks and nu-wave folk music, and in 2020 in a more manageable, office-friendly incarnation. Even moustaches returned, especially in the fashionable gay community, at the start of this century's second decade. This time, rather than big and bushy, they were pencil-thin. More Clark Gable than Hulk Hogan.

But while a beard can be man's best friend, our hair can also be our worst enemy. And Covid-19 only increased the potential number of reasons why. As the pandemic first took hold, there were a number of reports on whether beards presented a problem with the wearing of face masks. Facial hair could prevent a mask from sealing around the nose and mouth properly, undermining its purpose. Healthcare workers, in particular, were given guidelines by NHS employers in the UK; while in the States, the Centers for Disease Control and Prevention published an infographic with illustrations of 36 styles of beard or moustache highlighting which were mask friendly or which were not. The Van Dyke, English,

Fu Manchu and Garibaldi were all given big red crosses. The horseshoe, you may be relieved to learn, was borderline: you just had to be careful it didn't cross the seal. Those who had beards for cultural or faith reasons were consulted and offered alternative protective equipment such as helmets and hoods.

Other problems arose, too. There was a study published on the National Library of Medicine's website in 2018 that claimed "bearded men harbour a significantly higher burden of microbes and more human-pathogenic strains than dogs". Basically, men's beards have more bacteria than dog fur. In response, Amesh Adalja, an infectious disease doctor with Johns Hopkins University, told National Public Radio in America: "There's no evidence that having a beard per se makes you more or less vulnerable to the coronavirus. But you need to be really meticulous about the hygiene of your beard."

Whether the fashion for facial hair survives coronavirus or not, the follicles elsewhere on our bodies will continue to delight and dismay us. As we age, hair disappears from where we want to keep it – on our heads – and re-emerges, uninvited, elsewhere: ears, nostrils, shoulders and wings. What you have to accept from an early age is that hair is very much like children. Some hair will leave home as soon as it can and you'll barely get a call at Christmas; other hair will hang around for far longer than you wanted and make a mess; the rest is like unwelcome stepchildren that turn up later in life and expect you to treat them as your own.

Nose and ear hair

The step-hairs are the ones that sprout from your ears and your nose. And these become more prominent as you approach your fifties: one oddly long and dark strand of hair that suddenly peers out of your nostril halfway through a lunch as if it fancies a bite to eat, for example; the small tufts of hair that look as if baby hedgehogs have nestled in your ears. These are two of nature's cruellest tricks on man. The fault lies with the male sex hormone, Dihydrotestosterone (DHT), an offshoot of testosterone. Initially, DHT is our friend, since during puberty it helps develop your penis, balls and pubic hair. Unfortunately, later in life it can let you down. It is DHT levels that you can blame for male pattern baldness and, as if that weren't enough, excess hair too. As you get older, DHT encourages your existing body hair to continue to grow and new hair on your body to start to grow (and thicker), yet somehow manages to keep your penis at exactly the same size. Darn.

Almost your entire body is covered in some form of hair. The only parts without it are the palms of your hands, your lips and the soles of your feet. Before you are born, your body has soft hair all over it, including your ears. Unless you are born prematurely, this mostly disappears before the outside world can judge you. And then as you grow, so do two kinds of hair: vellus, which is short and fine in texture and sits on your head, and terminal, which is heavier (pubes, underarms and facial hair). As you get older, all-too appropriately, it's the terminal hairs that tend to rule the roost, and the hair follicles in our noses and ears, in particular, seem to become more sensitive to DHT and therefore produce bigger, larger hairs.

Terminal hairs apparently have their uses, but they sound to me as if they've been cooked up by a public relations company. The hairs in your nose and ears will help keep dirt and disease away from your orifices, they say. The nasal hair argument I get, up to a trimmed point, but the ear hair uses I'm not buying. Firstly, before ear hair started appearing, I'd never suffered from ear colds; secondly, during the Covid-19 pandemic, we didn't have to wear ear masks or beanies; and thirdly, you don't sneeze through your ears. And if hair is so helpful in keeping out dirt, how come we don't get any big hairs there until later in life? I spent far more time crawling around in the mud or in dodgy nightclubs in my youth than I do now. It makes no sense.

As with many areas of male beauty, some men don't care about these uninvited hairs. Normally, I would applaud their lack of vanity, but with ear and nose hair I think it's remiss. I used to work with an exquisitely dressed colleague at a Sunday newspaper – all bespoke suits and polished brogues –who took pride in his appearance (fine head of hair cut regularly in Mayfair), his home (William Morris wallpapers long before they were fashionable) and his work (the arts pages), but he never seemed bothered with the nostril hair that could almost be mistaken for a moustache, or the dark fluffy clouds attached to his ears that made it look as if he was wearing old-fashioned headphones. When we were leaning forward together checking some copy on a computer screen, his nose hair would sometimes prevent me from being able to read. Eventually, after we'd worked together for some years, I very politely brought up the subject of his nose hair by asking him if it didn't annoy him, peeking out from his nostrils and tickling his upper lip. He just chuckled (I couldn't help notice that his nasal hair bounced up and down as he did so) and said that his wife was always telling him he should trim it (I guess she must be able to feel it when they kiss). He never did.

Some men and women like hairy men, like hairy backs even, but there aren't many online forums dedicated to the love of lustrous locks flowing seductively from nostrils and ear lobes. Although in South Asia, where ear hair is at its most prolific, it has its fans. Radhakant Bajpai, an Indian grocer in Uttar Pradesh, whose 25cm-long ear hair appeared in the *Guinness Book of Records*, said that he considered his long ear hair to be a symbol of luck and prosperity. Despite his wife's objections, Mr Radhakant was very proud of his ear hair and treated it regularly with a specially made herbal shampoo.

If, unlike Mr Radhakant, your new-found terminal hairs don't make you leap with joy, there are various ways of eliminating them, but I can't pretend that the processes and regularity needed are not an immense bore.

1. Nose and ear hair trimmers. For the odd nostril and ear

lobe hair, a tweezing is perfectly doable, if a little ouchy, but it will remove the hair shaft and prevent another one growing back for some time. But if dealing with density rather than loners, you are better off using one of the many battery-operated hair trimmers on the market. They're designed to snuggle in and do the business without causing any harm. It's alarming how quickly new ones reappear, so you'll need to keep it handy. It's also tricky to see with ears if you've nixed them all successfully, so you will ideally have a partner who will kindly tell you when it's trimmer time (hopefully not during sex).

2. Longer-lasting refuge can be found with waxing; perhaps safer for ear lobes than with nostrils. Waxing also removes the shaft and therefore provides a longer-lasting result than just cutting them. I went through a period of about six months visiting a salon to get my ears and the area just inside my nostrils waxed as I liked the fact it killed the evil hairs rather than merely tamed them. But it's another cost, another lunch break gone, and so the trimmer won. You can buy DIY wax kits for your ears and nose. But don't.

3. Laser hair removal. Although some men I know recommend it, because the results are permanent, laser hair removal is quite expensive, often requires a number of sessions before being effective and, I imagine, isn't especially good for your mucous membrane.

4. Turkish barbers. Get a haircut in any one of the growing number of Turkish barbershops popping up around the country, and part of the service at the end of your cut is singeing the hairs on your ears. A lit taper or wand is quickly and expertly wafted around your ears to burn off any unwanted fluff with remarkable success. Don't try this at home with a Diptyque candle.

A tip: I can never decide whether it's nature being kind or cruel that your eyesight fades (officially at the age of 46) just as these errant hairs start to appear. Is the eyesight failing a bid to save you the horror of seeing what's happening to your nose and ears, or is it just acting like a complete tosser? Trying to aim a tweezer at your earlobe while looking sideways into a mirror with a fibreglass spectacle arm in the way is no mean feat. It's worth investing, as I did, in one of those round 5 x magnification mirrors (go for the ones that sit on a stand rather than the ones you attach to a wall so that you can put them away if you've got guests). They're called make-up mirrors (mine even lights up) but you can buy them online from somewhere called plumbworld.co.uk and you can't really get anything more butcher-sounding than that.

Eyelashes

Eyelashes are good. Thick eyelashes accentuate your eyes and make them look more intense and broody. They also signify a healthy lifestyle. A lot of women find longer eyelashes on men attractive. And eyelashes, unlike nose and ear hairs, serve a purpose in an aesthetically pleasing manner: they protect your eyes from debris, dust and flying bugs. Some of us are born with naturally long and dark eyelashes; some of us with short, pale stubby ones; and many of us at some point have burnt half of our eyelashes off by pretending we knew how gas lighters worked when we were drunk.

If you're not entirely happy with yours, there isn't a whole amount you can do to change them without the use of cosmetics. And I'm afraid – a constant theme in this book, I know – you will shed more eyelashes once you hit your forties and fifties. Some claim that castor or coconut oil can help eyelash growth, but there's no proof that's the case. Nor is there with the many over-the-counter eyelash growth serums on the market. The most effective, by prescription only, is called Latisse in the US and Lumigan in the UK. It is manufactured by the same company that owns Botox. However, there can be a number of potential side effects – hair growth around the eye as well the eyelashes, pigmentation changes in the iris and itchy red eyes. For blokes, especially, I wouldn't recommend it.

Less permanent alternatives include eyelash extensions for men – watch the video on Buzzfeed – or false male eyelashes that you can buy via Amazon. But perhaps the easiest, and most readily available, option is an eyelash tint, which most male grooming parlours have on their service menu.

When I took over as editor of *Esquire* magazine many years ago, the team and I worked day and night for months redesigning the magazine from scratch. There wasn't much sleep involved. When it came closer to relaunch day, the company's publicity team lined up some press interviews for which I would also have to be photographed. I looked knackered, so it was suggested that I go and have a facial at a salon nearby to alleviate my puffy, red, sleep-deprived eyes. I told the beautician what needed fixing. "Have you thought about tinting your eyelashes?," she asked. I hadn't. "It will put more focus on your eyes themselves rather than the area surrounding them." "Are you sure it won't look obvious?," I asked her. "No-one will know," she assured me. "It will just make your eyes look a little darker and bigger." Win win, I thought. She did what she needed to do and I returned to the office 45 minutes later, confident that my colleagues would assume I'd just nipped out for a sandwich. "Bloody hell," said one, as soon as I walked through the door, "when did you turn into Joan Collins?"

Eyebrows

I'm sure not many of you will admit to having watched *Love Island*, fewer still *Geordie Shore* in the UK or *Jersey Shore* in the US, but if you have – or indeed snuck a peek at any reality show in the last couple of years – you may have noticed that the male eyebrow has been under severe attack. The bloke brow has been plucked, waxed or threaded to near extinction. These sharp-edged, thin-lined, surprised-looking eyebrows that feminise the face to an unattractive degree are now as popular with the lads as they are with the contestants in *RuPaul's Drag Race*.

While nobody wants eyebrows bushy enough to hang Christmas baubles from each December, there is surely a happy medium – especially as the shape and colour of your eyebrows can radically change your appearance.

Most of us know that we need to pluck out the odd stray hair (there's alway one strand that's a different colour to the rest, twice as long, and reaching out for help), that we need to split up mono-brows (despite the prices Frida Kahlo's work reaches at auction) and let the barber give our brows a little trim on occasion; what we don't realise is that a bit of overzealous peace-keeping up there can have warzone-like results: eyebrow hair often doesn't grow back – so be really careful how far you go.

Suzanne Martin is the expert behind many of London's most polished faces. Having worked for many years as a make-up artist with Christian Dior, she has spent the last decade focusing on perfecting eyebrows. Until recently, Martin's clients were all female, but men are now starting to come, too – mostly at the behest of their wives.

The reason is that a well-crafted eyebrow truly balances the face, says Martin. Too unkempt, or even lopsided – as men age they tend to lose hair on one side more than the other – and it will affect your entire face more than you imagine. Eyebrows that are too close can make you look cross, she says; too arched and you look permanently surprised. It's about finding the right balance – not looking too feminine nor too werewolf.

Tinting your eyebrows is another potential pitfall, warns Martin. There are really only three shades available over the counter and in most male grooming parlours, so getting the right colour is nigh impossible.

If you take your eyebrows – or lack of eyebrows seriously – Martin is known for her semi-permanent treatment that involves effectively drawing hairs, one by one, on your skin. More refined and less invasive than microblading (a tattooing technique), the effect is very natural, takes two painless 90-minute sessions to complete and has little or no downtime.

Martin drew on my eyebrows so I could see how they would look if they were fuller or a tad darker, as she would do with any client before progressing to the next stage. The difference was quite remarkable. It somehow appeared to pull my whole face up without making it look as if I had two hefty slugs crawling across my forehead. As with most approaches to grooming, it's more about enhancing what you have, rather than trying to create what you haven't.

I didn't need to have my eyebrows treated in this way, despite them being a little on the scanty side, because there are numerous other, less-high-maintenance ways to keep your eyebrows in shape.

If you're happy with yours as they are, then the occasional plucking out of stray hairs with a tweezer should do the trick. If they're a little wilder, and you're a little more nervous – or like me you wear spectacles and obviously can't see them easily when you take your glasses off – then head to a salon or barber shop and they will do it for you. If it's a unisex salon, keep an eye out to make sure they're not over-zealous. I occasionally get mine threaded: a process in which a line of hair is caught between a twisted double strand of cotton thread before being removed. It's an ancient technique that originates from India and the Middle East and has the advantage of being accurate, quick and painless. A happier alternative to waxing.

Finally, there are a number of new eyebrow products on the market that you may think sound unnecessary, but I promise there are two that are definitely worth a try. One: eyebrow gel combs. You brush the gel onto your eyebrows and it just pushes all the hairs in the right direction and stops them sticking out all over the place; just as you would with the hair on your head. It's quick, easy and effective. You'll notice how much smarter it makes your upper face look in a very subtle way. Two: eyebrow definers. Similar to the gels but they come with a dab of colour to make your eyebrows appear a teeny-tiny bit darker. Again, this gives you a bit more definition and a stronger-looking eye shape. Also, dark eyebrows can contrast well with grey or silver hair.

Back and shoulder hair

It's strange that while chest hair, despite going in and out of fashion (the Bond films are a good barometer of whether body hair is "in" or not), is always considered socially accept-able, and for many, desirable, poor old back hair has never come in from the cold. Why does the hair on the back of our bodies cause so much more concern than that on the front? If you are attracted to hairy men, what is it that makes the geography of that hair so important to you? You would imagine, too, that those men who have hairy backs wouldn't be too fussed about it since they'll barely ever catch a glimpse of the hair themselves.

Yet there is no doubt that when you're lying by a pool or on a beach and a fellow bather strolls past with dark fur on his back you can't help but take a second glance. Why? Man Has Hair on His Body isn't exactly headline news. Of course, as with most beauty goals, we've been conditioned by decades of advertising images and movie stars who often have had no hair at all on their waxed upper halves. These ingrained images have made us believe that back hair is unusual, a defect, something to be removed. And unlike almost every other element of traditional male physicality, back hair has never appeared in a favourable spotlight. Well, not for 40 years since the more hair-tolerant late 1960s and early 70s. If you rewatch the 1971 James Bond film *Diamonds are Forever*, there's a scene where Connery takes a phone call while in the bath and he clearly has hair on his shoulder and his back. And before that, in 1967's *You Only Live Twice*, when Connery is being bathed by Tiger Tanaka's giggling handmaidens, the head of the Japanese secret service tells Bond that they are all fascinated by the hair on his chest. "Japanese men all have beautiful bare skin," he tells him. Bond replies: "Japanese proverb say 'Bird never make nest in bare tree'."

Today it seems bird and bloke do make nest in bare tree. Apparently, 60% of 16–24-year-old British men regularly remove their body hair; it's a generation that's grown up with images of bare-torsoed football heroes like David Beckham and Cristiano Ronaldo posing in Armani underwear, hairless models like David Gandy, all shiny smooth, selling designer perfumes and Daniel Craig's Bond stepping out of the sea looking as if he had actually emerged from a giant vat of Veet.

In an age when, marvellously, men can choose to wear make-up once more (see 1980s and 18th century etc), skirts once more (see 1980s and 19th century etc), and can choose the gender they identify with (that's newer, but about time), then surely they should also be allowed to wear back hair, once more, without fear of being judged or ridiculed.

The truth, however, is that not everyone feels comfortable with back hair. And if they don't want to have it, for whatever reason, then they should have the choice and the tools to remove or curtail it. The methods to do this are pretty well known. The most obvious route is waxing. But it's not the perfect solution as it's painful, doesn't last as long as you'd hope and, however much aloe vera you apply afterwards, the chances are you'll come up in a rash. And as the rash disappears, the hair regrowth starts again. The other issue is that sweat irritates the newly bared skin. Most people want to bare their skin because they're about to head somewhere hot for a two-week vacation. Hmmm.

In my forties, I noticed small patches of hair beginning to emerge from the lower part of my shoulder blades (wings). They weren't especially visible, but enough to annoy me at the time. I tried waxing and thus the insight above. I had similar results when I tried a hair removal cream. And it smelt disgusting. You can also elect for laser hair removal, if the area isn't too large, but I couldn't be bothered.

I now, very occasionally, and before a holiday, use a hair trimmer to cut the strands down to near invisibility. I know, I'm too cowardly to be a positive body hair activist. While reaching your own wings doesn't sound that easy, there are tools that have been invented for just that purpose (if you don't want to ask your partner): DIY electric back shavers that have extendable and bendable handles to enable you to reach those far-flung bits with relative ease.

Pubic hair

Sorry, but it needs a mention. Especially as 69% of men trim their pubic hair, and 17% shave it off altogether. I think I was a late comer to this trend, only taking up manscaping duties down there once I reached 40. And only then because a stranger told me that everyone else did. I had been seeing a personal trainer, twice a week, in a small gym attached to a hotel near the *Wallpaper* magazine offices in central London. The gym was mostly for the use of hotel guests and its personal trainers; there were only a couple of men who trained themselves there. One was called Tim, a well-honed

German accountant, who also worked nearby. Tim would train at lunchtimes, which was when I had my sessions, and we would nod hello to each other as we were often the only two in the changing rooms afterwards. After some months, the nods turned into brief and polite chitchat. Tim was gay, it turned out, but had absolutely no interest in me other than a curiosity about my job. The world that *Wallpaper* covered – mid-century houses, fashionable destinations, global cuisine – was one he liked to ally himself with. However, one day, as I stepped out of the shower, Tim casually commented in his droll Germanic accent that I should consider trimming my pubic hair. As pleasantries go, it was a left-field approach. I looked down, at my not especially hairy pubic region, and felt a little lost for words. "Oh," was all I could come up with. Tim could sense my embarrassment. "I hope you don't think I'm being rude," he added, putting some wax into his hair, "but every respectable gay man should trim." He packed away his gym kit. "Goodbye. See you next week." Well, that was me told.

I suppose, having been married to a woman and fathered two sons before deciding to date men, I was a little behind on gay etiquette. I hadn't noticed that everyone was taming their pubic hair. I asked my friends – gay and straight – whether they kept an eye on down there and it turned out that a lot of them did. Ten years later, it seems to be the norm, as the statistics above clearly illustrate. And there seem to be two reasons why. One, as per usual, is because it's currently considered aesthetically pleasing; a trimmed pubic region is fashionable. In the same way that advertising models, sportsmen and movie stars all have trimmed body hair that better shows off their gym-honed bodies; Pornhub actors all have trimmed pubic hair that better shows off their sex-honed penises. Your manhood appears larger, appears to stick out further, if there isn't much pubic hair surrounding it.

Second, is that a trimmed pubic region gives the impression of cleanliness and hygiene; there's less stuff for bits and bobs to get caught up in. I don't know about you, but I'm pretty sure reason one has more influence than reason two. In fact, reason two isn't entirely factually true, either. Pubic hair is there to protect your genitals from bacteria and other pathogens, and to help when your crotch gets hot and sweaty. Pubic hair can also protect you from skin abrasion and rashes that could otherwise be caused by friction during sex. Our hair down there is more hygienic than it looks.

Most pubic hairs, incidentally, grow to between half an inch and one and half inches long. The reason for their curliness, however, is unknown. And, guess what, as you hit your fifties, and your testosterone decreases, so will the amount of hair you have down there.

After Tim's comments, and my straw poll of mates, I began to trim. Initially, with a small pair of scissors, and then, as I became more confident, with an electric shaver. Get the setting wrong, however, and a nasty nick can be both painful and unsightly. Balls are not easy to shave. Imagine Tim's face if I stepped out of the shower with a small piece of bloodied tissue attached to my bollocks. As well as avoiding injury, you need to avoid shaving off too much hair. You don't want to look like a teen bride or a member of some unsavoury cult. Nor do you want your nether regions to appear lopsided; as if your scrotum has had a stroke.

To avoid any of the above mishaps, an increasing number of men head to waxing salons to have their hair removed by a professional. There was even a trend at the beginning of this century for men to opt for "boyzillians" (based on the female all-off treatment, the Brazilian), where all the hair would be removed from around their penis and testicles. Personally, I think this looks a bit creepy on a bloke. More acceptable, if you are going to head down that route, is the traditional back, sac and crack wax. Here you will have the hair removed from your testicles, your back, as well as any hair on or in between your buttocks. Usually, a patch of hair, if so desired, will be left sitting politely above your penis. Obviously, since I can't bare (sic) missing out on almost anything, I have tried this myself. I had three intimate waxes over a period of a few months about a decade ago. Quite why it took so long to realise that this process was humiliating, painful and pointless, I'm not so sure.

This is how it works. The nice lady (or man; although they were always ladies at the salon I went to) introduces herself, leads you to a cubicle where she leaves you for a few minutes while you take your clothes off, lie on the table and place a towel over your waist. She then returns, heats up the wax while asking you about holiday plans – almost like a normal haircut – and then it's time to begin. Sac and crack waxing is a participation sport. You are given tasks to do. They tend to start with the bum; it's less painful and therefore a more gentle beginning. If your buttocks are being waxed, she will apply the hot wax to them, wait a few moments and then tear it off when the consistency is right. If you have a very hairy bottom, I imagine this bit could hurt. I don't and so avoided this stage altogether. But then, humiliatingly, you are asked to either go on all fours or just stick your bottom in the air. It feels very wrong mooning the poor beautician but it is, at least, at her request. To make the process easier – and this is the bit that makes you wish you were dead, or less vain, or less hairy – she asks you to pull your butt cheeks apart so that she can apply the wax between them without anything getting in the way. You then remain in this very vulnerable position for what seems like hours (while hoping she's not taking a picture for Instagram Stories) until she is ready to strip the wax off again. Physically, it's mildly uncomfortable; mentally, it's torturous. But at least quick. Once your bottom is smooth and free of wax, you turn over for her to do the same thing to your testicles. This time you hold up the shaft of your penis to keep it out of the way. The pain as the wax is torn off your balls is tear-inducing; it's horrific. It's so bad you are not even embarrassed; you are merely furious at the hand that life has thrown you. You hate everything and everyone. You even hate your penis. Briefly.

The whole process, including adding some soothing gel and powder to the stripped area, and a few minutes to recover before getting dressed again, takes around 40 minutes. You then head back outside with a slight tingling sensation in your pants and a sweaty feel between your cheeks where there is no longer any hair. It's odd. The next day, unless you're unlucky and develop a rash, there is something quite pleasing about your newly sculpted region; your tamed topiary; your Tim-friendly lower facade. But, for me, it didn't prove pleasant enough to do it more than three times. Ultimately, the pain wasn't worth it. And since barely anyone would see it apart from my partner at the time and myself, what was the point? Much easier instead to rely on a specially designed pubic hair trimmer. These, as far as I'm aware, are relatively new to market, and have been created to ensure that a nasty nick on your bottom or balls is nigh impossible. Hooray.

Armpit hair

A random one, I know, but you should keep an eye on your armpit hair, too. Don't shave it off; it's very useful – it prevents friction between your arm and torso and retains scent to attract (or put off) potential partners – but the occasional trim might be advisable if yours tends to become long and straggly. Ideally, when your arms are down at your sides, tufts of hair won't peer out from under your arms. The hair should remain, anonymously, within the armpit triangle.

Incidentally, for men and women who suffer from excessive sweating of the armpits – hyperhidrosis – Botox is sometimes offered as a treatment. If stronger anti-perspirants or prescription tablets don't work, Botox injections block the nerve signals that tell the glands to secrete sweat. Some celebrities have Botox injected into their armpits before awards ceremonies so that they don't get photographed with any sweat stains on their outfits.

Men's loo rules

While we're having this frank discussion about our intimate parts, I will share the following advice. Whether in a public or an office loo, men's urinals contain as many conundrums as they do germs. Some of the rules, thankfully, are learned when you are still at school: don't look at your neighbour's willy, don't engage in unnecessary conversation, give it a shake at the end whether you need to or not and at least pretend to wash your hands afterwards. I can't remember what age I was when I was first confronted with a urinal. At first meeting, they can be quite intimidating. My friend Stephane was first sent to boarding school at the tender age of six. His mother, a nurse, and without a husband, felt she had no choice but to send him to school so that she could earn a living. After his mother had unpacked his trunk, made up his bed and kissed him goodbye, Stephane had to quickly learn how men and boys lived. He'd never met his father and so this new world was a complete mystery. He went to the loos and had a wee in a toilet in the cubicle and then tried to wash his hands in the little wall sink for children; much easier to reach than the higher sinks that he assumed were for the older boys. But no water came out. He studied it for a while, confused, and then gave up. Later that afternoon, when more pupils had arrived, he went to the loo again and decided to see how the others managed to make water come out of the little sink. To his disgust, the boys all peed in them.

As you get older, and more confident, you become less self-conscious about peeing with someone standing right next to you doing the same thing. Although sometimes, usually with no good reason, your penis refuses to pee. You stand there with your willy pointing pointlessly into the urinal without releasing a drop. Of course, you then become self-conscious that the person next to you has become aware that you're not actually peeing. You begin to wonder if he thinks you're just there for the ride, like a pee-vert. Even worse is when your dry spell induces a dry spell in the person next to you. You're both all too aware that neither of you is actually doing anything purposeful. The dilemma then, as in a spaghetti Western in reverse, is who will be the first to put their pistol back in its holster and back away from the urinal. Who will win and live to pee another day?

Fast-forward to adulthood and things don't necessarily become easier. The etiquette of having a wee in the office loo, in particular, is fraught with danger; you soon become aware of a complex and hierarchical system of acknowledged behaviours and grunts. This became especially evident when I began working at a national newspaper. Newspapers, particularly in the mid-90s, were macho environments that thrived on in-fighting, factions and stress. This atmosphere leaked from the main offices into the bathrooms. Here were some of the rules I learned from my decade there:

1. Don't chat to the person next to you unless they are a close colleague; and even then don't feel obliged to make small talk.

2. Do not glance, even if the person won't see you, at your neighbour's penis. Even though there's a strong chance you have no natural desire to look at his penis, there's a cruel trick of nature that sometimes, without your say-so, makes your eyes do so anyway.

3. If your neighbour farts at the urinal next to you, you have to pretend either to not care or not to have heard it. Do not, under any circumstance, jump in fright or giggle.

4. If, after standing at the urinal for around 20 seconds, you have not managed to urinate, admit defeat and back off. Any more and it might appear you're lingering unnecessarily.

5. Try not to fall asleep at the wheel. When I worked at the *Evening Standard*, the editor, who would arrive at the office at 5.45am each morning, would often nod off halfway through his pee, his head resting against the wall above the urinal. It was best not to try to wake him.

6. When you have finished urinating and are placing your penis back into your pants, let out an audible groan. The idea is to make a sound that lets the others at the urinal

know you are lifting a large and heavy object back into its place of rest.

7. Wash your hands with only a cursory glance in the mirror, if at all. Even today men will look embarrassed if you catch them looking at themselves. Except in gyms where they do little else.

8. Make sure you don't lean too closely on the sinks when you wash your hands. This could lead to an unsightly damp mark on your crotch. If this happens, you will need to retreat into a cubicle until it dries, or adjust your tie so that it hangs low enough to conceal the stain. Whatever you do, don't thrust your crotch into the hand-drying machine; this could be misconstrued by others walking into the toilets as inappropriate behaviour.

9. If you've been in a cubicle, it's impolite to flush and exit at the same time as the person in the one next to you. For a number of reasons, particularly if they were doing a loud poo, they may not wish to be recognised as your noisy neighbour. If it turns out to be your boss, it might be unsettling for both. Let him wash his hands and exit the room before you flush and leave the cubicle.

10. Always check your fly is closed and that there is no loo paper attached to the bottom of your shoes. Open-plan offices can act as a cruel catwalk.

Chapter 3

The Hair on Your Head

AS AN 18-YEAR-OLD, ONE A LITTLE too happy to experiment, I already knew there were limits with hairstyles. But back then I still decided to ignore them. And the fault for that lay with a 1980s pop group called Duran Duran. The band's "new romantic" outfits of disarmingly baggy trousers, white flouncy shirts with puffball sleeves and ornate cropped jackets topped off with unsmiling pouty lips and tinted bouffant hair were, I felt at the time, ones to be emulated; especially that of the keyboardist, Nick Rhodes. I wanted to be Nick Rhodes. He got to stand behind his synthesiser pulling absurd faces and occasionally plonking his varnished fingernails onto a note or two. He was also a talented "artist". *Blitz* magazine published a feature about Polaroids he took of his telly with the colour button turned right up so that it looked all fuzzy and arty.

In my final year at a Catholic boarding school in Suffolk

(run by a religious order of De La Salle brothers), I decided that I would cut and colour my hair to look just like Nick Rhodes's: backcombed and tufty-tall on top, long at the back (a sort of elegant mullet) and sides swept back with a heavy application of S-s-s-Studio Line gel. Nobody at school had yet dyed their hair, so it would be a daring act of rebellion. But my bravery had its limits. The conundrum was that I would need to show the hairdresser at the ladies' salon in Ipswich a picture of Nick Rhodes's hair for her to copy, but I was too embarrassed to let her know that it was Nick Rhodes's hair. It wasn't especially cool for a teenage boy to admit he was a massive Durannie during a period when the band was mobbed mostly by screaming girls, not boys, across the globe.

But, ha, I came up with a clever plan. I borrowed a small pair of scissors and cut out a picture of Nick Rhodes from *Smash Hits* magazine. I then – and this was the genius part – cut around the hairline so that it was no longer attached to Nick's face. This wasn't easy, as his hair was wispy, spiky and dangly to cut around. But eventually I had a small piece of paper in the shape-ish of his hair. It resembled a flattened spider. I carefully took the piece of cut-out paper to the hairdresser and asked her if she could give me the same hairstyle. She held it in her hands and studied it, without smirking, kindly didn't point out that even with my clumsy cutting it was pretty obvious whose hair it was, and preceded to give me a pretty accurate Nick Rhodes haircut. I couldn't afford to pay for it to be coloured and so had to do that myself back in my room at school. Luckily, when you reached the sixth form, you were given your own room – with a sink. Sinks were used for brushing your teeth in the morning and as urinals during the night.

The colour I'd chosen from Boots, within my budget, didn't quite capture Nick's expensive combination of highlights, frosted tips and textured shades of blond and tawny. It didn't even capture blond, as depicted on the packet, as I had been too nervous to leave it on for long enough. Instead, I emerged with a head that was a flat, rather iridescent orange colour. I looked like a Berocca.

Appearing from my room with orange hair which, after it had dried, now resembled a startled Basil Brush, caused quite a stir. The new romantic trend hadn't really reached Ipswich, and certainly not my Catholic boarding school, and so everyone touched and stared and commented as if they were at a petting zoo. Inevitably, I was soon called into the housemaster's study to explain my actions. Brother Richard calmly reminded me of the school dress codes, admitted it didn't mention hair colour but said that he would be amending that shortly, and asked why I had felt the need to change the hair and colouring that God had given me. Newly emboldened by my pop-star looks, I told him that it was a form of self-expression, and that Christ himself was a bit of rebel. I was also tempted to point out that Jesus had "dyed" on the cross to save mankind but couldn't work out how to emphasise the different spelling. Brother Richard suggested I go home for a week to work out with my parents how to "amend" my unchristian hair.

I couldn't face the palaver of dealing with my mum's displeasure, or my drunken stepfather, so I pretended to Brother Richard that I'd gone home but actually went to stay with my friend Emma, a day student (girls were allowed in the sixth form). Emma had very understanding parents; they didn't bat an eyelid that Nick Rhodes had grown on the top of my head. Emma's father instead made me watch *Les Enfants du Paradis*, a new-wave black-and-white French film that featured a beleaguered mime artist called Baptiste that he said looked like me. Baptiste's hair looked nothing like mine, especially as there was no colour, but after politely watching all three hours and ten minutes, I decided I didn't want to look like him. Her dad's ploy worked, and the next day, I agreed to get my hair recut: off went the spiky bits on top, chop-chop went the dangly ones at the back. Emma's mum then dyed what was left dark brown. Instead of Nick Rhodes, I now looked like Marc Almond. I wasn't best pleased, but was at least allowed to return to school and sit my exams.

But my inner new romantic hadn't disappeared; it merely lurked patiently inside of me. My appearance had tasted freedom; it had learned that, with a ridiculous haircut, change of clothes and inane expression, I was able to turn into someone else. Emma's dad was right; I was more like Baptiste than I imagined.

I discovered that the way I looked could change how I felt; this in turn could change who I thought I was. Just as in the *Mr Ben* cartoon series from my childhood, in which a mild-mannered, bowler-hatted man would go to a costume hire shop, try on a different outfit in the changing room and then enjoy a relevant adventure as this new persona – for example a fireman or safari hunter – a new life was only a change of clothes or haircut away. As David Bowie sang in 1977: "We can be heroes. Just for one day." All you had to do was go into the changing room.

Whenever I write a piece for *The Times* newspaper that's looking at the tricks and treatments available to those who wish, or can afford, to fiddle with their appearance, it's often fun to look at the comments posted underneath the piece when it has been published. Some of *The Times* readers who find the time to comment on these stories tend to be rather furious that I've written about such a flippant subject; so furious, in fact, that they've found the time to read it all, log on and write a comment. For example, posted below a piece on what a hair transplant entails: "What a joke. Worrying so much about one's hairline. Is it an attempt to distract from problems elsewhere?"

In some ways, to some degree, perhaps these commentators are right. In my case, worrying about my receding hairline may well have stemmed from my obsession with everything looking as perfect as possible; a lifelong quest to create calm from the chaos I experienced in my childhood. But perhaps it's also the simple fact that I would look shit with no hair. Most bald men look great; it suits them. Look at Bruce Willis, Dwayne "The Rock" Johnson, Vin Diesel or Jason Statham – they all get to play handsome heart-throb action heroes. Neither has being bald done Jeff Bezos much harm. Me? Not an option. When I was in my early thirties, and everyone seemed to be cropping their hair, I decided to give it a go, too. It would be a lot less hassle each morning if I had a buzz cut. My wife thought it was a good idea, and that it might really suit me. I went to the barbers in Soho to get a number one cut, she went to the shops, and we arranged to meet in a cafe 45 minutes later. I got there first, with my newly shaved head, and sat in the window with a coffee. When my wife walked past and saw me sitting there, she was so shocked at how appalling I looked that she walked into the glass door without opening it first. There was still a smudge of red lipstick on the glass when we left 30 minutes later. At work the following Monday, my colleagues were equally aghast. "Oh no, you look really ugly with no hair," they sweetly pointed out. And they were right. It was pretty obvious from that moment on that I should try, as hard as I could, to hold onto my hair for as long as possible.

The one thing most men seem comfortable talking about when it comes to their appearance, apart from the grumpy trolls on the *Times* website, is their hair – or lack of. It's the bit of us we're allowed to be vain about... but only up to a point. We can safely point out that our hair is thinning, grey-ing or gone altogether, but suggest a cure and everyone looks a little uneasy. I was at a dinner party recently and the men, mostly spurred on by their wives, admitted that they'd goog-led hair transplants. The host even fetched a can of spray-on hair to everyone's amusement (it looked like fuzzy felt), but none of them had properly looked into taking Propecia or other hair loss treatments (or so they said), nor had anyone actually gone to visit a surgeon to find out more. So if you're like them, at a (hair) loss as to what do, here's the beef.

There is no doubt that the thought of a transplant can be quite intimidating: the cost, the pain, the time off work. And then there's the dilemma of how long to wait before having one, where to get it done. Go online and you'll find plenty of stories and pictures of successes and failures, disastrous trips to Turkey and an endless fascination with celebrities who may or may not have had one.

The Times once asked me to interview a Harley Street hair surgeon about the concerns that men typically experience when considering a hair transplant, and to get him to give my hairline his expert opinion as part of the piece, too. Rather more quickly than I hoped, he pointed out that my hairline was now quite high (despite my having a fringe) and that in an ideal world I would bring it forward an inch or so. He reached for a marker pen and drew an outline of how it could look. Ahhh, the perils of seeing what could be… three months later I was back in his clinic, sat in the chair, about to undergo an FUE or, as I like to think of it, a hairline refresh.

Ultimately, there are two types of surgery: Follicular Unit Transplantation (FUT), also known as strip surgery, as it involves taking a thin strip of skin with intact hair follicles from the "safe" or "permanent" zone at the back and sides of the head (preferable if larger graft numbers need to be achieved); and Follicular Unit Excision (FUE), which involves extracting follicles individually from the back and sides of the head. This is a less invasive procedure, although you will need to have the back and sides of your head shaved and the hair density in the donor region will obviously decrease.

The procedure, to my surprise, is quite painless. A local anaesthetic is used and the only thing that hurts is watching the hair being shaved from the back and sides of your head. I looked like Kim Jong Un (or Kim Old Un, as a friend kindly pointed out). Since the transplant took about seven hours, I was placed in front of a large TV screen and watched the entire first season of *Peaky Blinders* while devouring a large bag of Haribo.

For the surgeon and his technicians, however, the process is quite intense. First, they remove the follicles from the back and sides of the head, one by one. In my case, 1,792 of them. The follicles are then trimmed, counted and sorted under the microscopes. After that, the surgeon cuts tiny incisions where the follicles are to be placed (again, you feel nothing, but the dull crunch-like sounds were a little off-putting) and inserts them individually. It's incredibly labour intensive. Meanwhile, all I was doing was sitting there as if I was in an episode of *Gogglebox*.

At the end of the procedure, I'll admit that I wasn't looking my best. My head was mostly shaved, the recipient area was a little bloody and swollen and I had clingfilm wrapped around my forehead to prevent infection on the taxi ride home. But there, peering out at me, was a new hairline made up of small follicles that a few hours before had resided elsewhere.

The trickiest part of the process is the aftercare. You will need to take a week, ideally two, off work. I'd booked my operation at the start of a fortnight's vacation in August. Initially, you need to protect the areas operated on from infection, be extremely careful with the fragile new grafts (you use a neck pillow at night so you don't rest on them), take painkillers and anti-inflammatory medication for a few days, and regularly use a saline solution to keep the grafts moist. It's pretty full-on for the first five days, but easily manageable. I even had some friends to stay during this time, although you have to avoid alcohol. After about a week, it all calmed down and, aside from a severe short back and sides, there was little clue to what I'd undergone. Two weeks later and I was back at work. The hair at the back of my head had grown enough to hide any signs of where the follicles had been removed, and my fringe hid the small new ones nestled at the top of my forehead.

After two to three weeks, the transplanted follicles fall out. It then takes about three months for the new hairs to start to push through again. After six months, the new hair growth was pretty impressive and, although shorter, had begun to meld in with the longer hair I already had on top. After a year, which is when I am writing this, it looks as if it has always been there, although it apparently takes 12–18 months to reach its full length and density, so is likely to continue to increase in thickness for a while still.

My hairline, while rejuvenated, didn't look incongruously youthful. And if I hadn't been so impressed with the results that I readily told anyone who would listen how amazing the whole process was, I could have perhaps got away without anyone knowing what I'd had done. Admittedly, the area being restored for me was relatively small and thus the transformation less immediately obvious to others. Larger areas will involve more grafts, more time, and be more transformative, and thus more obvious.

It's also worth noting that if you're having a transplant when you're relatively young (25% of those who experience hair loss will see the first signs before the age of 21), the chances are that you will face further hair loss and may require another transplant in the future. By the age of 50, 50% of men will have some form of visible hair loss; by the age of 60, it will affect around 66%. So the later you leave it, the better.

A good hair surgeon – and really make sure you do your homework or, even better, go with a personal recommendation – will be able to advise what can realistically be done now, what to expect in the future, and also what will suit you. Some men have their hairlines brought too low and look like the friendly one from *Planet of the Apes*; others have a hairline put in that doesn't look realistic (just too perfect), or appears too feminine. As with all these treatments, ideally you shouldn't veer too far from what was there before.

I wish more of the men who lament the loss of their hair could know how palatable getting some of it back again can be. It's odd, considering 80% of men experience male pattern baldness, that we don't share advice and experiences with each other more. Our family and friends are the people who should be able to advise us whether or not we should treat it, and if so, how. Admittedly, not everyone can afford it – it costs between £4,000 to £9,000, depending on the number of grafts.

Another way of fighting hair loss – especially if you catch the motherfuckers trying to run away at an early stage – is medication such as Propecia. And even after a hair transplant, you are advised to take it to prevent further loss occurring.

Propecia is a product that was released onto the market in 1997. It is the brand name for finasteride, which works by reducing levels of the hormone dihydrotestosterone (DHT) in the scalp: DHT contributes to male pattern baldness, and the medication helps to reverse the hair loss process by decreasing the effect of DHT on the hair follicles. In studies, 80% of men taking finasteride held onto their original hair follicle counts and 64% experienced some regrowth after two years of continued use. In the US alone it has 10 million prescriptions, including one, I'm afraid to say, for Donald Trump.

Others, I know, are against Propecia as it has a number of potential drawbacks.

One is that once you stop taking it, the hair you've held onto with its use will fall out. So if you want to keep your hair, this is a lifelong, not inexpensive, commitment. Second, in some cases those taking Propecia – about 3.8% –

can experience erectile dysfunction, loss of libido or smaller ejaculations. Sometimes these symptoms can persist even when you've stopped taking the medication.

Finally, there is the much-debated question as to whether taking Propecia, manufactured by Merck & Co, in 1mg doses can lead to depression, even suicide, in some patients. While research continues, and lawsuits are filed, doctors are advised to keep a close eye on patients and to take them off the medication if they do develop signs of depression.

What isn't in doubt is that the percentage of those who experience adverse reactions is very small, but the risk is still there. I've been fortunate enough not to experience any symptoms during the time I've been taking it.

The non-surgical alternative for those wishing to curtail hair loss without risking Propecia is Rogaine (minoxidil). It's been available over the counter and without a prescription in most countries since 1998 and has no known serious side effects, apart from a reported toxicity for cats. Most cats will, fortunately, be unable to reach the counter at pharmacies.

Minoxidil, initially developed to treat ulcers (unsuccess-fully) and then high blood pressure (successfully), comes in the form of a foam or drops that you apply, twice a day, to the affected areas of your scalp. It's believed to be most effec-tive with the area around the crown; and not of use to treat a receding hairline. Minoxidil works by partially enlarging the hair follicles (it's a vasodilator) and lengthening the growth phase of your hair, thus giving you more hair coverage. This means, of course, that it won't bring back hair in areas that are already bald. And alas, like Propecia, it stops being effective when it's no longer used. A number of men use both Rogaine and Propecia to combat their hair loss.

Oddly, given that I've fought so hard to keep hold of it, I don't care what colour my hair is. I just consider myself lucky to still have some. And I'm not convinced colouring ever works for men. Dyed hair on guys tends to look flat and unconvincing. Women can get away with it because they can introduce highlights and lowlights which give it depth and definition. Most men can't go down that route. I can always spot when someone has dyed their hair, especially if it's with a home kit, but if you're really not keen on the salt-and-pepper hair you're cultivating, or have gone completely grey – both of which, I think, always look great – then obviously its best to see a professional colourist first. Otherwise, there are a number of home dye kits designed to target only the grey hairs on your head.

To be honest, if you haven't used a home kit before I don't recommend it. During lockdown, I volunteered to dye my hair grey for *The Times*. The brief was, in the early stages of the social distancing rules, when hair salons had been forced to close and many pharmacies were selling out of hair dyes, to explore how easy it was to do it yourself. While some aspects of the ageing process have clearly been most unwelcome, I've always looked forward to having grey hair. My dad went silver at a relatively young age and I always thought it looked, if not quite up to George Clooney's standards, rather smart.

The local supermarket in Windermere, in the north of

England, where I now live, had a limited offering in the hair products section. Reading the back of the boxes, it seemed I would first need to bleach my hair peroxide blond with one kit, and then dye it grey with another. You have to wear special plastic gloves (we've all got used to those anyway, I suppose), apply a bleach solution (the ammonia in it smells horrid) and then sit in a chair for 30 minutes watching the colour literally drain out of your head. Afterwards you rinse thoroughly, add in a toner (to help play down the yellow) for 20 minutes and rinse again. Voilà. I was now bleach blond. Alas, instead of looking like a Californian surf dude, I looked more like the lovechild of Donatella Versace and Iggy Pop. I quickly unpacked the grey hair dye. This time I had to dab petroleum jelly around my hairline to prevent the dye staining my skin, apply the colour, wait 45 minutes, rinse, apply a conditioner and wait another 20 minutes. Time for the great reveal. Oh. Iggy was still with us; no sign of the silver at all. I stared in the mirror and Joe Exotic stared back at me.

What seemed vaguely amusing at 11pm after a few glasses of wine was far less so at 8am on a bright summer's morning with a work-related Zoom call booked in for 5pm. I FaceTimed my friend Louise, a hairdresser, who lives nearby, for advice. She screamed with a mix of laughter and horror. Obviously she was unable to come to the rescue in person, but said that she'd leave out a professional silver-grey hair dye mix in her front garden that I could pick up when I went for a run. I've never jogged so fast and with so little complaint. There was something reassuring about the potion she left out for me; it somehow looked more professional than the home kits I'd bought at the supermarket. I felt optimistic. Once again, I went through the whole rigmarole, washed my hair and peered into the mirror. It had worked. I was silver-haired (but with a slightly annoying yellow undertone if I'm honest). But I was now less Tiger King and more Sun-In King… or Gandalf the Gay as a friend cruelly commented (again) when I sent him a snap.

Chapter 4

The Eyes Have It

SITTING AT HOME, DURING THE FIRST lock-down, staring at my computer screen while waiting for endless Zoom or FaceTime video calls to start, there was always a slightly weary-looking virtual receptionist staring back at me. Initially, he looked as if he was enjoying his new role but, as the months passed, and his hair grew longer, and beard more straggly, and forehead more furrowed, it appeared as if he might be ready to risk an air corridor holiday to Spain.

Covid-19 had been devastating, globally, in so many ways – health, livelihoods, economies, families and social groups had all taken an immeasurable hit, while… on a micro level, some of us also questioned the way we look. Not only because many of us had to spend months glued to our Macs, our faces hovering at the top right-hand corner of a computer screen (until you eventually realised, months later, you could switch that bit off), but also because we hadn't been able to rely on anyone outside our households for help with haircuts or beauty treatments; we'd been unable to visit the dental hygienist or hit the gym. And, if you managed to hook up with Ocado, snacks were much easier to grab at home than they were in an office. Some of us found this immensely freeing (and fattening); others less so.

Whether you spent time during lockdown on Facebook and Instagram, or reading the papers and listening to Radio 4, you noticed that woven between reports on social distancing, furlough schemes and the hunts for a vaccine, was endless advice on how to cut your own hair (YouTube videos), colour it (spray-on cans), set up a home spa ordered from Amazon, shove chewing gum in gaps where teeth have fallen out, and dress up for virtual dinners or quiz nights where only your top half was visible to others. Television presenters filing their reports from home and office workers attending screen conferences would wear shirts and jackets while sporting only sweatpants and slippers off camera. Only a few made the embarrassing mistake of getting up for the bathroom mid video call while wearing just a pair of skimpy underpants or, in one case I saw online, nothing at all.

Of course the virtual receptionist staring out of my screen during lockdown was me. And, I have to admit, I didn't particularly warm to him. I would sometimes spend large chunks of video calls – the boring ones, at least – pretending to be fascinated by what everyone was saying, but in reality just staring at the strange little me on the screen. This pastime didn't fill me with joy; I didn't look at myself and think:

"Phwooar! I'd give him one." But neither did I recoil. I just couldn't avoid focusing on the parts of my face that bothered me the most; especially the areas of skin around my eyes – with or without a mask on, they seemed to be pleading for help. Or perhaps just a good night's sleep…

Endless well-meaning articles and books have been published about the importance of sleep for your health and well being. Getting a good night's sleep is a sleepless task for many of us, whether that's due to stress, working patterns, light pollution or a debilitating medical disorder such as sleep apnoea. For the one in three people who suffer from insomnia, reports that a lack of sleep can lead to obesity, heart disease, high blood pressure and diabetes don't ease the mind. I haven't slept properly, unaided, for years. As soon as I hit the pillow, exhausted and ready to sleep, my mind will cruelly remind me of everything I forgot to do that day and need to do the next day, and drag up every mistake, faux pas and missed opportunity I have buried in my subconscious over the past 20 years.

I have tried natural remedies (peepo, still wide awake); sleep clinics (gave me nightmares; better than nothing, I suppose); podcast serials (can't sleep because I need to know how the story ends); giving up booze (no help, but did give me more energy); and meditation apps such as Headspace (I tried the one where the narrator languorously describes the inside of an antiques shop on a rainy Saturday afternoon – alas, I was bolt upright, dying to know if they had a Georgian oak console table at a good price). So every night for the past eight years or so, I have had to take a prescription sleeping pill to help me to put my mind on pause for a few precious hours. Not ideal, of course, and even with that help I never get the recommended seven-plus hours.

A less severe, but still frustrating side effect of sleeplessness is looking knackered. (Google any prime minister or president's eyebags before and after office and you'll see what I mean.) While a lack of sleep should be taken seriously and the cause dealt with as soon as possible – not easy when many sleep physicians advise more holidays and less stress and you're in the middle of a pandemic – it may be a comfort to know that there are a few tricks that can make you appear more rested than you feel.

Speak to a lot of aesthetic doctors today and they will tell you that "looking as if I've had a good night's sleep" is what most of their male clients ask for.

One of the more extreme measures for treating the area around your eyes is something called TotalFX laser treatment. Rather than fix eyebags (btw, despite what you might read, pile treatment creams don't do the trick), this laser treatment is designed to correct the crepey, slightly saggy skin you can get under the eyes and tighten the lids that slightly droop above them. Basically, TotalFX consists of two procedures. The first element, called DeepFX, involves a narrow laser microbeam – a pocket-sized version of the one that nearly castrates Bond in *Goldfinger* – which is used to remove columns of tissue through several layers of skin. Why? To stimulate collagen production, which improves the appearance of fine lines, wrinkles and scars and tightens the skin up. Next up is the ActiveFX part. This involves a larger beam that targets the upper layer of skin to remove hyperpigmentation, encourage new skin generation and again remove fine lines.

A word of warning: always do a serious amount of homework before undergoing a treatment like this. And ideally speak to someone who has had it done before. You want to know about the person doing it, the clinic they work from, the risks involved, the real end benefits – and, where I slipped up with this one, the recovery time…

The procedure itself wasn't so bad. You sit for an hour with half of your face covered in a white anaesthetic cream, feeling a little self-conscious every time someone pops in to see how you are. Once the doctor is happy the anaesthetic has kicked in, the 30 minutes of laser treatment begin. You certainly feel the jabs of heat as the laser is applied, but it's no more painful than a pin prick. It actually feels like someone is spitefully holding a small pen torch to your eyelids. Some people have their whole faces treated in one go; I was happy we were only doing my eyes.

Afterwards you are given written instructions, plus anti-bacterial spray, special cleansing gel and Vaseline-like ointment to apply post-treatment. You are also advised to avoid sunlight for a few weeks, and after that use a high-level SPF cream. Back home, I looked in the mirror and it wasn't as bad as I thought. I looked sunburnt and my eyes a little swollen, but it didn't actually hurt.

But the next morning. Bloody hell. I woke up early, eager

to see what had happened overnight, to discover Freddy Krueger staring back at me in the mirror. My eyes had almost closed with the swelling, and the areas around them were red and oozing. Thankfully, it was a Saturday. I looked so appalling that, perversely, I couldn't help but laugh. I sent a picture of myself to a WhatsApp group of friends, asking if anyone fancied a night out as I wanted to show off my hot new look. All the replies featured a screaming-with-horror face emoji.

Fortunately, the face is quick to repair itself: 48 hours later, the oozing was replaced by scabbing (which made me look like one of the reptilian humanoids from *Dr Who*); two days after that, the scabs crumbled away to leave a raw-looking layer of skin. As the days passed, the redness paled to a mild baby pink. By this time I was back at work and my colleagues, although too polite to ask, must have wondered what the hell had happened. If I'd done my research properly back then, I would have booked at least a week off work to recover; ideally longer.

It actually takes at least three or four weeks to fully lose the pinkness. It's a long time; especially if you work in an office. Even longer is the time you have to wait to see if the treatment has worked: from six months onwards. I sometimes wonder if we're told it will take six months before the benefits show because cosmetic practitioners know that, by then, we will have forgotten what we looked like before and won't have a clue as to whether it worked or not. Or we will be so thrilled that we don't look like lizard man any more that any semblance of normality will be welcomed as miraculous.

The truth is that six months later, and beyond, there was a noticeable improvement in the skin around my eyes. The wrinkles and lines had faded (but not disappeared), the eyelids were perkier and the skin less crepey. My friends (begrudgingly) noticed the difference more than I did. About a year later, I received multiple compliments – and believe me, my friends are not like the kind insects in *A Bug's Life*. Would I recommend it? If you hate the area around your eyes, yes, but only if you can deal with a good month of looking rather peculiar. It's a tough call. I'm not sure I would do it again.

The other non-surgical treatment gaining traction for the living dead is Profhilo. This isn't a dermal filler, which tends to give people odd moon faces, I think, but a helpful dose of hyaluronic acid. Hyaluronic acid, which we produce naturally, is key to our skin remaining and looking hydrated. The Profhilo is injected into five areas of the face and, over the next 12 hours, dissipates beneath the skin, giving it a fresher, more dewy appearance.

The treatment stimulates four types of collagen and remodels the deep supporting layer of the dermis. It takes about 30 minutes, the needle pricks are a little uncomfortable, and you do look a little bee-stung in places for up to 24 hours. I had it done on a Friday afternoon and was shopping in M&S Food the next morning. And by the end of the weekend, for the first time in a long while, I looked as if I'd had a rather refreshing nap. The treatment needs to be repeated one more time, a month later.

Profhilo has become increasingly popular as an alternative to filler as it looks a lot more natural. The problem with traditional dermal fillers is that many people overuse them and their faces look bloated, or they use them to rid the face of lines that are actually attractive – such as those that help make your eyes twinkle, or the ones that form from the side of your nose to the corner of your mouth when you smile (nasolabial folds).

One treatment, using fillers, that has become increasingly popular with men is the jaw enhancement. If you have a weak chin, or your jaw isn't quite as firm or as square as you would like, a few well-placed injections of filler can sculpt it into the required shape. The results are immediate, the bruising (dependent on how easily you bruise) non-existent or short lived and, if you don't like it, you can reverse the treatment by having the filler removed.

I have an uneven jaw (my lower jaw is less developed than my upper one), which gives me a bit of a weak chin, so I tried this myself. A few jabs later and straight away my chin and jaw looked –subtly – more prominent. It felt a little sore for a day or so, any bruising I may have had was hidden by my beard, but the slight discomfort was overridden by the joy of my new-found macho jawline. I spent the next few weeks proudly stroking my new chin (a process that took a lot longer than previously) every time someone asked me a question at work. I'm not sure anyone else noticed the change – unless I asked them – but that wasn't the point. The point was that I liked the change. And if it made me happy, then good.

Filler treatments tend to last around 6–12 months (see page 180 for more insight and facts on fillers) and aren't cheap so you've got to be sure they suit both you and your pocket. I didn't have my chin and jaw treated again after the first time as they didn't bother me enough to make it worth the investment. The Profhilo treatment, however, I've continued with.

Finally, the least invasive, and most cost-effective, way to look temporarily less tired is by using make-up and eye gel masks. Dozens of brands – men's and unisex ones – offer under-eye concealers, tinted moisturisers and eye gels and masks that help disguise dark areas under the eyes and blemishes, or reduce puffiness. The concealers and tinted moisturisers will obviously help by masking the appearance of the skin; the eye gel masks – you store them in your fridge – will cool the area around your eyes and reduce the puffiness. In my experience, there is very little difference in effectiveness between the products at each end of the price spectrum. Most of these, for the faint-hearted amongst you, come in packaging that looks as if might contain a screwdriver rather than a cosmetic so there will be no mark on your machismo.

Chapter 5

Brace Yourself

THE BRITISH TOOTH HAS LONG BEEN an object of ridicule; particularly with our transatlantic friends. The fact that we were late to the game with hygienists, whiteners, straighteners and veneers saw us caricatured over the decades as a nation of shopkeepers with wonky-shaped, yellow-coloured tusks; as exemplified by Mike Myers' Austin Powers character. But boy, has that changed. Faced with a constant bombardment of perfectly spaced, shiny-white gnashers on everything from the latest Netflix dramas – where even the cadavers have enviable grimaces – to more home-grown shows such as *Strictly Come Dancing* – the professional dancers have grins that light up like the Blackpool illuminations – there is no doubt that an aesthetically enhanced smile is no longer a taboo. And whether you're an avid selfie-taker or not, thanks to the rise of Instagram and other photo-sharing apps, we are less able to grin and bear it when our smile is evidently a little under par.

The problem for many of us, especially men, is that we want nice-looking teeth, but don't want to spend months wearing braces or slipping on teeth-whitening trays each night to achieve that satisfactory smile. Even Invisalign braces – the clear plastic ones that produce a quick effect, with little inconvenience – seem too much bother for some. Yet there is no doubt that a uniform set of teeth – on the right side of Hollywood white – can take 10 years off your face.

You've probably noticed a new breed of cosmetic dentists popping up on the high streets – you can hardly miss their pearly-white smiles – whose focus is not only improving the condition of your teeth, but the appearance of them, too. These smile doctors, as they've been called, have an array of quick-fix tricks and treatments that need only an hour or so of your time. Enter the reception area of one of these practices and you will see a clientele of fashionable young socialites, high-ranking politicians and familiar faces from TV. So if you've got a big party in 10 days' time, a wedding the next week (perhaps your own), or something interesting to say on a current affairs show, it's not too late to upgrade your smile.

If you are really in a hurry, the quickest solution – depending on the state of your teeth, obviously – would be to get a hygienist to use airflow polishing (jetflow, air and sodium bicarbonate) to properly clean them. This will help to remove plaque and red wine, tea and coffee stains. Ideally, you would then have an in-chair whitening treatment – four successive 20-minute cycles at a clinic – followed by a couple of days using self-administered whitening treatments. I'm afraid most over-the-counter home-whitening kits are pretty pointless, and not always good for your enamel or your gum health.

Joy of joys, with only an hour or so in a clinic, you can then opt for composite bonding (a form of veneer) to remould your teeth to look even, straight, whiter or shorter. (Who wants to look long in the tooth?) Basically, you have your teeth shampooed and conditioned before a modelling resin is applied to give them the form required. So if your teeth are discoloured, or you've ground them down, or your gums are receding, this can all be aesthetically altered in no time at all.

These quick-fix veneers are prone to chipping and can stain, so you will need the occasional MOT. As mentioned above, coffee and tea (tannins), red wine (the worst culprit) can stain your teeth, but so can soy sauce and curry. Rather a cruel assortment, as they're easily some of the tastiest items that appear on a menu. At least avoid them for the first few days after your teeth have been treated, as they'll be at their most porous.

And, if you can bear it, use a recyclable straw for drinking your coffee and tea as it will limit the amount of tannins that make contact with your teeth. Most coffee shops now provide paper straws at the counter, and you can readily buy reuseable ones – metal, glass or plastic – for exactly this purpose. I have a number of the latter that I now carry around with me. They're designed to be collapsible after use, and come with a pocket-friendly container. Initially, I felt a bit self-conscious about pulling out a straw to drink my morning coffee, especially in a big open-plan office, but have noticed that so many others are doing it now, too.

Less commonplace is using a straw to drink a nice glass of red wine; it does rather take the edge off a good burgundy. I did so a few times when eating in restaurants with friends, just to see their reaction, and it didn't disappoint; nor did the look of distress on the face of the sommelier when he saw me place a retractable straw into the tasting glass of pinot noir he'd just poured.

If you're looking for a longer-term fix then you can have laser contouring for uneven gums (heals in days and you can go straight back to work); or invest in longer-lasting porcelain veneers (these involve a bit more time and money). You could even indulge in some Botox if your lower lip reveals too much gum. And, of course, there's the aforementioned Invisalign braces.

I wish Invisalign had been invented in 1976. When you're at a boarding school, sharing a long open-plan dormitory with 23 other 12-year-old boys in tight rows of beds separated only by small wooden lockers, you soon become less self-conscious about nudity, bathroom habits and how you look. Everyone insults everyone and, on the whole, you roll with the punches. Mirrors are the inconsequential things above sinks that you don't pay much attention to. Life is happening at too fast a pace to find the time to stop and stare at yourself. Who cares? Even I didn't. Until my mum took me to an orthodontist.

Over the previous year or so, a couple of my front teeth had started crossing, and I had also grown a slight overbite. It was Mum, not me, who had become aware of, and bothered by, this fact. The orthodontist she found, despite his ornate waiting room and plummy voice, had no personal skills whatsoever. He was crass and uncharming, oblivious to how I might feel as he casually and pompously announced that I'd need to have four of my teeth removed and wear an elaborate brace system for 18 months. It was when he got out an example of the brace that I would have to wear that I pursed my lips together tightly. I would need metal fastenings attached to the upper teeth on each side of my mouth to which, for 12 hours a day, I would then hook a sturdy fabric strap that would stretch out of the corners of my mouth and fasten at the back of my neck. This would apparently pull the teeth back and allow more room for my squashed front ones. I was going to be made to wear a horse's bit.

When we left his office, I pleaded with Mum not to make me go through with it. I was happy with my crossed front teeth; maybe they'd straighten themselves as I got older? But to no avail. A few weeks later, the condemned teeth were pulled out, the metal fasteners attached with glue to the bereaved ones left on each side, and plummy orthodontist-man demonstrated how after each day at school I was to head back to my boarding house, clip on the straps, fasten them at the back of my neck and keep them on until the next morning.

No-one had ever seen anything like it. When I returned

to school, all my fellow boarders were gathered together and told that I had to wear a special brace each evening which, if tugged, could pull my teeth out. They weren't to touch it, and needed to be especially careful within my vicinity. Unsurprisingly, everyone looked in my direction with both sympathy and delight. I, of course, was mortified.

The first evening I had to put on the contraption, a few boys gathered around in the bathroom to witness the moment, as if watching an episode of *Springwatch*. I had to stand in front of the mirror to see what I was doing. "Blimey," said Stamp, whose family owned a farm in Suffolk, "you look like a combine harvester." There were sniggers, and then one boy started singing, "Oh, I got 20 acres and you got 43. Now I've got a brand-new combine harvester and I'll give you the key." It was a song by the Wurzels that had been number one in the pop charts the year before. The boys soon ran off, distracted by the sound of someone's skateboard outside, and left me staring in the mirror at a face that, until a few months before, I'd thought was okay when I'd bothered to actually take a look at it. The experience with the orthodontist was probably the first time I became aware that how you look can let you down; that even a face can make mistakes.

Narcissus had stared at his own reflection and fallen in love with the beauty he saw in it. I stared at my own reflection and saw a piece of farm machinery looking back at me. I think it was from that moment on that my relationship with mirrors became a little unhealthy. Reflections were where you spotted imperfections.

Three years later, at the same school, with the brace gone, my mum inadvertently struck yet another blow at my attempts to remain on equal footing with my fellow boarders. It was 1980, I was now a sensitive 14-year-old, and Pink Floyd's anti-education single, "Another Brick in the Wall", had just been a huge hit. Naturally, it's rebellious lyrics had put the album it came from at the top of every schoolboy's wish-list. There was an excruciating tradition at school that on your birthday, after breakfast but before lessons, everyone would gather around your bed and watch you open all the gifts and cards that had been sent to the school. Twenty-three pairs of eyes would be peering enviously at you. If there were edibles, you would have to share them with all the boys there; if the pile of gifts was sparse it was humiliating; and if the choice of gift was deemed inappropriate you could count on it being mentioned, frequently, for many months to come.

I was relieved when I spotted that the wrapped gift from my mum was the shape of a record sleeve. I had dropped enough hints that I wanted the Pink Floyd album. As I tore off the blue-and-white wrapping paper (featuring cross-eyed penguins for some reason), the boys around me nodded to each other in anticipation of spotting the now familiar glossy white album cover featuring black-outlined bricks and a scrawling red typeface. Except, all too soon, and to my incalculable dismay, it turned out that it wasn't Pink Floyd's *The Wall* at all. It was the original West End cast recording of the musical, *Annie*. Instead of a pile of bricks on the sleeve, there was a little girl in a red dress with big curly hair.

Orphan Annie sprang to mind once more as I was finishing this book. I went to the dentist and asked if she could repair my chipped composite veneers. She said that in all truth they would continue to chip as my overbite (that pesky overbite is still there after all these years) meant that my bottom teeth kept pressing into, and damaging, my upper ones – and the veneers fixed on them. She said it would be worth my while visiting an orthodontist first to see if they could sort the overbite. One appointment later and it has been recommended that I sport fixed ceramic (train track) braces for between 18 and 24 months. Braces. Again. In my fifties. I mean. Tomorrow, tomorrow, I love ya' Tomorrow. You're always a day a way.

Chapter 6

Vanity Flair

AS A GENDER WE HAVE TRAVELLED through the last few decades with appallingly fragile egos; we're terrified of getting something wrong and yet equally appalled at the thought of asking each other for help. We're both suspicious of, and competitive with, men who we feel look better than ourselves.

When I spent four years as the editor-in-chief of *Esquire* magazine in the UK, an inordinate amount of time would be spent trying to choose and secure the "right" celebrity to feature on the cover. The cover, after all, was the magazine's billboard; the image that would hopefully catch the eye of potential readers browsing through the shelves at newsagents and lure them into the world of *Esquire*.

It was hard not only deciding which celebrity would appeal to readers, but also persuading the chosen celebrity's public relations team to let you photograph and interview that celebrity. The publicists, on the whole, were charmless Rottweilers whose worth was proved by how unhelpful they could be at every point and turn in the process of fixing up a flattering cover shoot for their client. Sometimes the weeks of late-night calls to these monosyllabic monsters was worth it when you finally saw your cover with George Clooney or Brad Pitt peering out from amongst your neon-coloured coverlines looking as if butter wouldn't melt in their mouths.

One month, *Esquire* decided to dedicate the magazine to style icons of the past and for the cover, instead of photographing a Jake Gyllenhaal or Christian Bale, chose a selection of movie heroes such as Paul Newman, Steve McQueen and James Dean taken in their heyday. They turned out to be some of *Esquire's* best-selling issues ever. The team sat down and tried to analyse why: was it their achievements or authenticity that made the punters part with a fiver to buy an issue of the magazine that month? Or was it the fact that they were dead? Perhaps the readers felt more comfortable carrying around an issue of a magazine that featured a bloke who was no longer alive, or a threat. "Yep, Paul Newman may be more stylish and better-looking than me, but I've still got one up on him, mate. I'm breathing. Beat that, Newman."

We rarely ask other guys outside immediate family where they got their blazer from, their hair cut, or for advice on how to wear a certain style of trousers. This inability to discuss anything sartorial is the reason that, until recently, entire generations of men have dressed clumsily. Thank God today for the web with its how-to videos and what-they-wore stories enabling men to check out what others are wearing without being seen to do so; they can ask style or grooming questions from a search engine, knowing that their conundrum will remain anonymous. When I was working at Mr Porter, the men's e-commerce site, the most popular stories we published online each week were ones such as Five Ways to Wear a Navy Blazer, or How to Clean White Sneakers. Do I wear a black bow tie with a navy tuxedo? Alexa has the answer and she isn't going to judge.

Of course there are men who enjoy discussing clothes and appreciate quality and design. But even with them, until recently, there were limits. The open admiration of what men wore was often merely a game of one-upmanship disguised as an appreciation of the finer things in life. Think of the 1980s and its bullish Wall Street status stamps such as pinstripe suits, contrast colour shirts and vivid red braces (Michael Douglas as Gordon Gekko); the scene in *American Psycho* where the rival stockbrokers battle over business cards, like a game of Top Trumps, salivating over the raised lettering, watermarks and bone-coloured card. In the 1990s, showing off got easier still when even off-duty symbols such as underwear, jeans and luggage were plastered in a riot of indiscreet logos. Today, in-your-face has been replaced by in-the-know. The story behind what you wear has become the acceptable face of men's fashion; a swing from showy to stealthy – i.e. knowing the thread-count of a Loro Piana poplin shirt, the cashmere sourced from Inner Mongolia that goes into a Brunello Cucinelli sweater, or the craftsmanship behind a bespoke shoe last created at George Cleverley.

But there is no doubt that what you choose to wear – even in the age of video conferencing and virtual dating – can make you, or the person you're meeting, feel at ease in every sense. Our choice of clothes can be used as a form of defence (battle dress), comfort (sartorial Xanax) or energiser (try a sharply tailored blazer or a box-fresh pair of white sneakers). Clothes were used, pre-avatars, to help you create the persona you wished to project. Now avatars on gaming sites do that for us. Ironically, a host of gaming sites enables you to buy virtual designer clothes to dress your avatars with at vast expense. Some futurologists predict that in the not-too-distant future most of the interactions we have with each other will be through our avatars and not our real selves... I can't decide whether that is good news or not.

Although it may not always seem so, dressing well, or socially acceptably, is within the reach of most of us today. Menswear in particular is relatively undriven by rules and diktats; you can wear sneakers whether you're 17 or 70; geography no longer controls what's available to you; and style inspiration is on offer to all via an effortless scroll or swipe. Dressing today is dictated less by trends, dress codes and commutes and more by comfort and self-expression. We have become a nation of armchair connoisseurs.

But despite this, there are still a few tips and insights that don't always get shared by men with each other; or that only become apparent with experience rather than research. And, having listened to readers' and customers' concerns and

questions over the decades that I've worked at men's magazines and men's e-commerce stores, I'm going to share a few
of those conundrums, along with some mostly helpful, and
occasionally spiteful, solutions.

Size and fit (for purpose)

Fortunately, most of us have by now come to terms with
what suits our body, our personality and our environment.
If we're lucky, we're happy to embrace whatever these may
turn out to be. If we fight them, the chances are it could
be a messy and protracted brawl. But like a tinted moisturiser or a regular haircut, there are a few failsafe pieces in the
conventional male wardrobe that will nearly always come to
your rescue whatever the occasion, even in times of crisis.
When suffering from a hideous hangover, for example, the
following items of clothing will nurse you through the day as
effectively as a Solpadeine and a bacon butty:

A well-cut navy blazer

A blazer is the modern man's armour; it readies you psychologically and physically for the bar or the boardroom. A good
blazer steels your resolve by straightening your shoulders,
puffing your chest and pulling in your waist. And navy is
one of the most flattering colours to wear against your skin
(as you get older, always wear navy and not black; the latter
drains colour from your complexion).

A crisp pale-blue shirt

If your hangover has left you feeling crumpled and looking wrinkled, the freshness of a well-pressed pale-blue shirt will help straighten you out.

A patterned tie

Although there are fewer occasions these days when a tie is deemed necessary, a strong tie – especially with video calls when only your top half is visible – will distract from the pain on your face. With everyone working more from home, and formal occasions less frequent, the tie could be another item on the list of everyday pleasures the pandemic has killed off. Although if we removed everything not entirely necessary from our wardrobes, there would be very little left indeed.

Smart shoes

If you're not stuck in front of your computer, then put on a smart pair of formal shoes. At least your footwear, if not your presentation, will be polished when you're hungover. Shoes are apparently one of the first items of clothing a woman will notice when she first meets you. When I was at Mr Porter, we sold more footwear than any other item of clothing. You would not believe how many pairs of shoes or sneakers the average man would buy. I often wondered if it's because the size of our feet are one of the few sizes we are able or willing to remember correctly.

As well as knowing what suits you, you also become more

convinced as you age – not always with good reason – about what you believe suits others. Sometimes you subconsciously resent other men for being able to wear items of clothing you clearly cannot; at other times an item of clothing can conjure up a memory or even a sound that almost repels you. I have three of these:

Three style items to avoid:

Deep V-neck T-shirts

Since we moved out of London, my husband and I have found ourselves frequently playing host to city-dwelling friends who fancy the idea of a boozy Saturday night dinner followed by a sleepover and a lazy Sunday stroll before nipping back to town. The things I enjoy the most about this are: a) seeing how everyone looks first thing in the morning when they stagger down to breakfast (as it's my home I always have more grooming remedies to hand than they do), and b) noting the diverse array of slumber-wear that appears at a house party.

The most popular choice for first thing in the morning is the sweatpants and T-shirt combo. This seems perfectly sensible as it will see you through breakfast and, if you're so inclined, it will work, too, when teamed with wellies and a jacket for a potter outside. The most popular styles I see are grey jersey sweatpants, hoodies of a more adventurous shade and, I'm sorry to say, an inordinate number of low-slung, V-neck T-shirts.

Oh, why oh why, is the deep-V T (no coincidence it sounds like a sexually transmitted disease) so popular? Every time I ungraciously point out to my guests how unappetising these look on men, they stare back at me as if I'm some mad old uncle (Monty). I suppose they have a point. But most of these V-necks are so low they morph into a Y-front. I imagine each time they go to the loo, wearers pull the V down a little lower, pull out their willy and have a wee without any need to touch their underpants at all.

I just don't think men should wear tops that have more non-top than top. I don't want a pair of someone else's pecs, however toned, to land on my muesli as they reach over the table for the milk jug; surely sideboob displays belong to red-carpet film premieres, not Sunday morning brunch.

Flip-flops

There is no doubt that flip-flops are a practical holiday choice: cheap to buy, light to pack, easy to wear and wholly waterproof. But, they have a major flaw: the very sound that has given them their name – that grating flip-flop noise that, in full flow, makes me want to scream. The sound of cheap rubber repetitively smacking against calloused heel is not a pretty one.

My reaction may sound a little extreme, but flip-flops and I have history. As a fully-fledged fashion student with all my cash spent on new outfits to parade in the three different nightclubs we religiously went to every week, my grant would usually run out three weeks into the new term. After I'd not eaten for months, and been turned down for a Saturday job at Liberty, there was only one way to earn some extra cash: prostitution.

I rang two dodgy numbers for escort agencies I found in the back of a porn magazine and offered my services. Humiliatingly, they weren't interested in my sending a photo in, let alone granting me an interview. I must have had a very un-escorty telephone manner. I tried one more number, this time trying to sound like an East End plumber, but still no luck. I obviously didn't sound very sexy at all.

Desperate, and hungry, I was told by a friend about a hospital near London Bridge that paid people to be guinea pigs for new drugs being trialled by the major pharmaceutical companies. You would have to stay at the hospital, for a few days or a week, in special dormitories with a random group of hard-up students, backpackers and fashion victims; some of you were given the drugs, others fed placebos. You didn't know who got which.

We would all have to eat the same food, sleep the same hours, have regular blood and heart tests throughout the night and not leave the clinic under any condition. I did two drug trials as a student, although I can't remember what they were for. I do remember being offered one trial, which paid a lot more than the usual ones, but it involved stopping your heart briefly to see if the drug they were testing would kick-start it alive again. I sensibly decided no Yohji Yamamoto jacket was worth potential heart failure.

Anyway, the reason I mention this is that while locked

in these over heated hospital clinics, populated mostly by Australian gap-year students, there was nothing to do but watch daytime telly, read a book and listen to, yes, the click-clack of flip-flops. All anyone wore in these places were baggy shorts, polo shirts and blasted flip-flops. So when I look at those harmless pieces of foot-shaped rubber, I don't hear the sound of gentle waves and shifting sand; I hear the theme tune from *Neighbours* and a tannoy announcing it was time for another injection.

Asshole scarves

Queuing up politely to buy a coffee and a jelly doughnut in a bustling café in Montauk, New York, two summers ago, I got to the front and ordered a flat white from the elderly lady behind the counter. While she went off to make the coffee, another elderly lady asked me if I wanted anything else. "Yes please," I said. "Three of those delicious-looking doughnuts." When the lady with the coffee returned, and saw someone else was getting the doughnuts for me, all hell broke loose.

"Sir!" she shouted extra loudly so everybody could hear. "That is not fair!" Pardon me? "That is not fair. One helper per person. We are busy, sir!" She then turned to face everyone in the queue and everyone in the café and yelled once more. "Okay. We have a problem here!" All eyes turned to me and glared.

The problem was I should only have been helped by one person. Two people helping me with my order – even though that help was proffered, not requested – was deemed a crime of monstrous selfishness. Of course, I was mortified. As I sheepishly carted my coffee and doughnuts (they weren't all for me!) past the long queue at the door someone muttered: "Asshole!"

This tragic episode clearly left its mark, as soon afterwards I bought and read an entire book about assholes by an American philosopher called Aaron James. In *Assholes: A Theory* (Doubleday), James looks at what makes an asshole, and how to handle one, so to speak. There are many types of asshole to be found – more often male than female, the book says – but there is one particular type of asshole he describes that seems especially prevalent in the fashion world: the Delusional Asshole. Aaron James describes one of the main traits of the Delusional Asshole as an inability "to pick up his reflection in the eyes of others, from what is evident to all".

I'm sure for you, as with me, a few names spring immediately to mind. Occasionally, however, we may fall into the delusional dressing category. A survey in the *Daily Mail*, for example, included a list of what women don't like to see men wear. Not all of which we might have been aware of. Some of the choices were obvious: men in socks and sandals, Ugg boots, Lycra, or baggy grey sweatpants (good luck with that one). Others on the list were a tad more controversial: low-slung V-neck T-shirts (told you), trousers with elasticated hems (I have a pair of those), pink jeans (a bit harsh) and girly scarves. Effectively, the ladies who were polled for this survey thought that these garments made men look like assholes.

The question of scarves is an interesting one. Especially now that men opt to wear winter scarves and summer scarves. I'm not exactly sure what was meant by "girly scarves" – that seems rather inappropriate terminology today – but I imagine they are referring to one of two things: either the fashion for summer scarves in which flighty bits of fabric are worn loosely and pointlessly around the neck, or the recent penchant for tying perfectly reasonable woollen or cashmere scarves in ever more elaborate ways and places.

There has been a puzzling trend for scarves to appear on parts of the body far removed from the neck – scarves worn around trousers as belts; around chests, making the wearer look like some over-embellished Napoleonic general; or wrapped around necks so many times he resembles an Ancient Egyptian mummy on show at the British Museum. Sometimes it's a fine line between looking cool (or, in this case, warm) and just looking like a bit of an asshole. According to Aaron James, an asshole is made, not born. So hold back a little on your scarf arrangements. And on the number of servers that help you with your doughnut and coffee order.

Four items that can go nicely right or horribly wrong:

Sweatpants

A piece of clothing I tried to resist for years was the sweatpant or tracksuit bottom. Initially, I agreed with Karl Lagerfeld, who once said, "Sweatpants are a sign of defeat. You lost control of your life, so you bought some sweatpants." But, unlike Lagerfeld, sweatpants are still with us, and today I understand why. It was about 2015 when the fashion for sweatpants seeped out of the sportswear category and infiltrated the more formal zones of our wardrobes – cue grey sweats teamed with heavy black brogues, button-down white shirts and navy blazers – and it seemed as if the classic trouser was heading for extinction. A bit like the onslaught of the grey squirrel, the grey sweatpant was fast becoming a superior species, forcing its dandyish rivals to retreat to the back of the closet.

The appeal of the sweatpant is one of contrasts. It was invented in the 1920s for athletes, then adopted in the 1970s and 1980s by the hip-hop community (most famously, perhaps, by Run-DMC), and from there its appeal grew and travelled across the globe. The fact that British prisons then made the grey sweatpant standard uniform for new inmates only helped enhance its street appeal.

And the sweatpant has held its own ever since. It has survived an attack by the onesie; ignored the fact that the matching top-and-bottom look is also standard wear for small toddlers needing easy-access nappy changes; and smirked at nightclubs who refuse entry to those wearing a pair. For an item of clothing to gain such wide generational appeal, for quite so long, there must be more to it than mere fashion, and a reason many high-end designers sell luxury cashmere versions at corresponding expense, season after season.

My only concern is that for an item of clothing whose origins lie in skilled athleticism, they emanate inertia. The century following their invention – despite the popularity of gym classes, yoga and athleisure – has seen the energy wrung out of them; a danger now more pressing than ever since so many of us can wear them "to work" in our new home offices.

All that said, I have to confess I'm an avid wearer. As are my sons. And, clearly, pretty much everyone else. And these are my theories as to why:

1. Look around you and you'll see that many sweatpant wearers are not off-duty Olympians, or on their way home from a rap battle. They like pulling on their sweats each morning because they require little effort (no belts or zip), the waistband happily expands as you dig into your builder's breakfast or lunchtime pint and you can bung them in the washing machine and not give them an iron. I think it's the "no-brainer" part that has a lot of appeal. Today, we all work extremely hard to keep up with the demands of work, and the demands of how everyone expects us to look (at work and play). Meanwhile, our working hours – home office or not – are for many the longest they've ever been. This means that not only is our leisure time shorter than it has been for years, but we're actually too knackered or brain-dead to make the most of it. Thus, the idea of getting up and dressed before the coffee has brewed on a weekend morning is much less

taxing if all the clothes you slip on kind of match, don't have complicated fastenings and are likely to fit despite the size of the takeaway you gobbled down the night before. We now do ready-made convenience dressing that complements our ready-made convenience foods.

2. There is currently less onus on us to get dressed to go out. Ironically, because of lockdowns or the internet, a lot of our social life is virtual or solo. You don't need to get dressed to go to the supermarket or the record shop (food from Ocado, music from iTunes). Want to catch up with your friends? No need for a trip to Starbucks to say hi, just click the "Like" button on their most recent Instagram post or join a Zoom call. Fancy a date, or a shag over the weekend? Forget bars or clubs, just swipe through a few mugshots on Tinder or Grindr. All this is done from the comfort of your sofa, in the comfort of your sweats.

3. This is possibly the most controversial of my theories and, although you may publicly argue otherwise, privately you will know I'm right. What do most of you do when you're at home, lying on the sofa watching telly? Whether you realise it or not, you're putting one hand down inside your pants and fiddling with your willy. I'm not sure why: maybe because it's warm down there, maybe it's because you like to make sure your willy is still there, or maybe it's some sort of pet substitute. Some longtime married friends came around for supper the

other night, and the subject came up. The women were all resigned to the fact that their husbands, without a second thought, would happily spend their evenings on the sofa with a hand down their pants having a friendly fiddle. Some were so absent-minded about this habit that they would inadvertently do it even when they had guests. (Beware hosts handing out crisps is my advice.)

It's time I finished. It's tiring typing with one hand. But at least my other one is all warm and cosy.

Cagoules

Cagoule is one of the least alluring words in the men's style lexicon. Nobody thinks, "Ooooh I'm going to put on my lucky cagoule before I go out tonight." Neither do you want to be friends with the sort of person who says, "Don't forget to pack your cagoule for the awesome stag party I've planned for this weekend." Nor have I noticed many of the designers at London Fashion Week describe their signature style as "cagoule".

The problem is that, despite its unsexy name – cagoule sounds like something a toddler says when its nappy needs changing – this item of clothing is pretty essential if you're holidaying in the UK (which more of us who live here are having to do). Cornwall or the Lake District are popular with passing showers throughout the summer months. This dilemma is particularly pertinent to me as I've just moved to the latter. With its rugged mountains and plethora of lakes, the Lake District is as lovely as it is for a number of geo-graphical reasons, the main one being that it rains all the time. As the train heads north through Cumbria, I stare out of the window at the beleaguered families on their annual holidays shuddering on wind- and rain-swept station plat-forms, barely recognisable as human since no sign of bare limb or facial feature is visible through their shapeless, drip-ping wet clobber. Some of those poor holidaymakers spend their entire week's vacation sleeping in wind-battered tents or caravans lodged in water-soaked fields.

You might wonder why I've moved here. Well, in the moments of good weather the Lakes are blessed with, there is nowhere more breathtaking. I bought an old farmhouse half-way up a mountain, miles from anywhere, so that I can go for weeks on end ignoring all my own advice in this book as nobody can see me. The conundrum, even when I'm tucked away up here, is the cagoule word. I don't want to look like a member of Oasis or Keith from Mike Leigh's *Nuts in May*.

Luckily, there are now a number of brands who've tackled the waterproof-clothing problem without veering too near cagoule territory. Instead, you can call them shell jackets or field jackets. Windproof, waterproof, breathable and light-weight with sealed seams, they've made it possible to stay dry and look fly, even in the rain.

Also beware any of the above that feature too many pock-ets. You need pockets when venturing into the great outdoors to hold your phone, a Cadbury's Twirl and air freshener, of course. But some shell jackets have so many things to open, you could confuse them for an Advent calendar (indeed, after a few weeks' wear, many of the pockets may contain a surprise). Waterproof hiking trousers have also been given the multiple-pocket treatment, with openings all over the front, back and sides. Just give yourself plenty of time to find the right one when you want to go for a pee.

Biker jackets

How do you get away with wearing a black leather biker jacket? We know how good they can look: cast your eyes over Marlon Brando in *The Wild One* (1953); or Alex Turner in the Arctic Monkeys' video for "Why'd You Only Call Me When You're High?". Even Depeche Mode's Dave Gahan still gets away with wearing a black motorcycle jacket and he's nearly 60. On me, well, they just don't work; I tend to look like an extra from *Lovejoy* (1986–94) or, even worse, *Cruising* (1980).

I optimistically once swapped half a London flat for a leather jacket. I bought my first apartment, with a mate, straight out of college at the height of the late-1980s property boom. After spending a large part of my £11,000 annual salary doing it up, I sold it a couple of years later as boom turned to bust and, after repaying the mortgage, I got back a paltry £1,200. I was so pissed off I went straight to Prada and spent it on a leather jacket identical to the one Tom Cruise wore in the first *Mission Impossible* film. I still have it and yet have only worn it once in all that time – since you ask, it was to a goth club in Islington called Slimelight. My button got accidentally caught up in a girl's cobweb top and took a good five minutes to untangle. By the time I was free again, I discovered that my mates had left the club; they thought I'd pulled. I suppose I had, but not in the way they thought.

I'm sure you look much better in them than I do. What it comes down to, as is so often the case with clothes, is frame of mind. If you have the confidence, or the conviction, that you suit a leather jacket, then the chances are that you probably do. It's when you start to feel self-conscious, or a fraud, that it all goes Pete Tong (or Freddie Mercury, in my case).

Sadly, I'm aware – and clearly have been for some time – that I'm not really a rebel without a cause, that I look more natural sitting astride a horse than a Harley, and that I will always look like a former member of St Joseph's College Chapel Choir than one of the Libertines.

But the leather jacket is a menswear classic that never truly goes out of fashion and so, if you're not in the cast of *Rumble Fish* (1983) – I'm keeping you on your style movie reference toes – and are popping to the shop for some pitta bread rather than heading out to fight a rival street gang, just how do you make one work for you?

Choose a leather jacket without too much detailing on it. Leave the bells-and-whistles versions for the real bikers. The plainer the design, the easier it is to wear. Try teaming yours with a pair of coloured cotton trousers (a deep-green hue will work well), a crew-neck sweater (a flecked number in grey or navy with a bit of texture perhaps) and finish off with a pair of chunky black leather boots.

Otherwise, a leather bomber jacket is always a safe bet. They're a little less obvious, not so rock'n'roll, and look especially non-rebel in a good chestnut brown, though try to avoid looking too like Martin Shaw in *The Professionals* (1977–83, yes! another vintage TV reference!). These look fine worn over almost everything, but are particularly dashing teamed with dark skinny jeans, a matching polo neck and a pair of brown suede desert boots.

Ultimately, of course, if you've done your homework you'll head to US brand Schott, who designed and produced the first leather motorcycle jacket, the Perfecto, in 1928 (originally sold for $5.50 at a Long Island Harley-Davidson dealership; Brando wore a Perfecto One Star in the afore-mentioned film). The New York-based company also produced the leather jackets worn by all US military services in the Second World War, and later was a favourite of leather-clad punk rockers throughout the late-70s and 80s. With the Perfecto, you'll be wearing a leather jacket with a history of rebellion even if you're actually teaming it with a safe pair of chinos and a cable-knit sweater – more "mild one" than "wild one". Who's for a nice cup of tea?

Knitwear no-nos

Come rain or shine, there's always knitwear. Sweet, harmless knitwear. Or is it? Each season's knitwear comes with its own dilemmas.

When winter bites, it's hard not to covet all those triple-ply cashmere pullovers, cable-knit cardigans and voluminous crew necks in mohair and angora. But as much as you want to touch and snuggle up in them, there's a big problem with chunky knits. An inherent problem, really – and it's that chunky knits make the wearer look, well, chunky. In fact, whatever your waistline, however minor or momentous your moobs, most of the covetable knitwear at the moment will make you look like a great big fatty boom-boom.

I recently fell in love with a striped cashmere cable-knit cardigan that I stared longingly at online for weeks and weeks. But when I eventually ventured in-store and tried it on, tragedy struck. Instead of David Gandy, I looked like John Candy. And I'm a 32in waist and 38in chest. I can't work out who the guys are who are able to wear these gargantuan items of knitwear and not look like someone peering forlornly out of a beer barrel.

The other knitwear trend I've tried to embrace, with little success, is the polo neck. In theory, these are a marvellous idea: not only do they keep your neck warm, worn with a jacket they render a tie unnecessary, plus they have a healthy hint of 1970s Bond villain. The reality: they make your head look like a rather-surprised boiled egg. And, if you've got sensitive skin like me, give you an uncontrollably itchy neck.

My final knit pick of the season is the woollen beanie. Why does nearly everyone but me look good in one? I've tried wearing a big baggy one that hangs off the back of my head, a tight-ribbed one that fits snugly, and something in between the two. But no. Whatever I do, I end up looking like an unattractive extra from *Fargo*. I was relaying this problem to my ex-wife, who kindly and succinctly solved the problem: "You're too old." Oh.

So if you want to wear something knitted, what's the smart and stylish solution?

I think the trusty old V-neck doesn't get as much of a look-in as it deserves. The V-neck had some bad press a decade or so ago and it has taken a while to recover. Some think V-necks are an item only dads wear to match their Farah slacks (they are); others are still reeling from the memory of Michael Douglas wearing a V-neck with nothing underneath, while throwing a few uncomfortable moves on the dance floor with Sharon Stone in *Basic Instinct*. But, worn well, a V-neck will add a layer of colour into an outfit; fit snugly under a blazer it will negate the need for an overcoat. And, if you pop over to Milan, you will see how well the Italian men carry them off: not too baggy, made from cashmere or merino wool, in either a delicate pale blue or lilac, or a chic grey or camel. My favourite combination is a crisp, pale-blue cotton shirt worn under a school-grey merino wool V-neck with a navy wool sack blazer. Yum.

Talking of yum: please note that if you get a V-neck that fits well, it can be far more forgiving regards lumps and bumps than just a shirt can. If I've not convinced you about V-necks, the shawl neck is a stylish alternative. These look pleasing worn over a button-down Oxford shirt, or a plain white T-shirt for the weekend. If you pick the right one – especially in cardigan format – it can look smart enough to wear for a work meeting, too.

Don't underwhelm in underwear

About two decades ago, when I was the editor of a weekly style magazine, I published a column called Lucky Pants. The idea was that each week we would ask celebrities to let us photograph their favourite underpants and tell us why they liked them.

You will be surprised to hear that this was a short-lived column. However, the first celebrity to participate was the marvellous Michael Winner. The film director-turned-food critic agreed to send in a pair of his pants to photograph on the condition that we returned them within 24 hours and didn't forward them to *Private Eye*. When the package arrived, I cautiously opened the envelope and pulled out a pair of large but pristine white cotton Y-fronts. Not a career highlight, I must admit.

Winner aside, most men don't feel the need to air their underwear in public. Indeed, in 2007, when Jeremy Paxman wrote to Sir Stuart Rose, then head honcho at Marks & Spencer, to complain about the lack of support in the gusset of the company's underwear, he was dismayed that the correspondence was made public. And when asked whether he was referring to boxer shorts or Y-fronts, he refused to be drawn. He did say, however, that "when I've discussed this with friends and acquaintances it has revealed widespread gusset anxiety".

You imagine that most men don't discuss underwear conundrums over a pint in the pub. And until the last decade

65% of men's underwear was actually bought by women – for men. But times, and pants, are changing.

Step into a department store today and you'll see an overwhelming selection of underwear styles that didn't even exist until relatively recently, everything from boxer briefs to midways to pouches (eww).

One man who will happily discuss underpants with anyone who asks is Sacha Rose. He is the managing director of Derek Rose, a successful British heritage brand that started as a nightwear label in 1926 and eventually added loungewear and underwear. Rose has to keep up with what men want from their underpants, as well as how they, er, use them. And this involves discussing the finer points of our nether regions with both friends and strangers.

His extensive research has uncovered some interesting points. Most men, it turns out, don't use the fly in their pants when they go to the loo: they either pull the waistband down at the front or hitch one leg up to get to where they need to get. So first of all there is no need for buttons on flies (although Rose has introduced magnetic ones on his so we don't have to fiddle about too much).

The majority of men now buy their own underwear. As a gender, we have become more interested in taking charge of our appearance, although, unsurprisingly, the primary deciding factor is comfort (fabric, fit and quality), followed by price, packaging and brand name. And despite the popularity of boxer shorts – made fashionable in the 1980s after they appeared in the infamous Levi's jeans launderette ad –

the brief is the most popular style of underpant, says Rose, closely followed by the boxer brief (a hybrid of the two; a sort of clingy, jersey boxer). The reason for the brief's popularity is support (Paxman was clearly not alone when he worried about his gussets), especially with more of us participating in sport and gym workouts. Another consideration is that the formal clothes we wear now tend to be a lot more fitted, and a baggy pair of boxer shorts might cause unsightly lumps and bumps.

So how do we decide which style to choose? Apart from inadvertently catching sight of a colleague's undergarments in the changing room or subscribing to FansOnly, we have to base our decisions on the slightly in-your-face photographs of moody hunks with unrealistic bodies and pointy pounches that are constantly posted on Instagram.

Are we supposed to believe that we, too, will look like that if we buy a pair? And do they all have socks stuffed down their fronts? Rose says that some brands do indeed use pouch-enhancing objects or post-production wizardry. According to another source, David Beckham, who in the past has happily posed in his underpants on giant billboards for Armani and for his own range for H&M, apparently needed no help whatsoever in that department. If this is true, you would have thought Victoria could smile more often.

My 34-year-old brother-in-law says that he has never seen the point in buying new underwear until the current article falls apart. His last girlfriend disagreed, however, and told him to smarten up his act. He duly went out and bought 10 pairs.

According to Rose, most men bulk-buy their underwear; it's something we still look upon as a task to be got over with rather than a treat, perhaps. And what about the women he spoke to? What style do they prefer to see men wear? "Fresh and new is their main criteria," Rose says. "And some wives prefer there to be as much fabric as possible," he adds.

You might think your choice of underwear doesn't matter because nobody will see it, but you would be wrong. What happens if you get hit by a bus and the medics need to remove your trousers? What happens if you spill a hot drink down your leg and have to remove your scalding chinos in the middle of the office? What happens if you get lucky on a night when you weren't expecting any action?

Whichever style you choose, do not get a size too small as you will be left with unsightly marks on your skin from the waistband. You may also hamper any chance of procreation. While white underwear can look clean and fresh, it is to be avoided if you consume an orange vitamin C drink each morning. Black or navy is a little more practical in that case. Novelty or patterned underwear is not recommended. This is one area of your body where you don't especially want to be seen as Mr Fun Guy.

Shorter trousers make longer legs

Have you noticed that come rain or shine, city or seaside, town or village, there's an increasing number of men who look as if they're about to go for a paddle?

They stride along purposefully, in an otherwise normal outfit, with trousers inexplicably rolled up to their ankles, often with no sign of a sock. Who knew that hemlines could rise and fall in the menswear world too?

This trend for less trouser and more ankle (or "mankle" as its detractors have labelled it) has been on the rise for a number of years. It started off as a high-fashion statement and has ended up as a more mainstream one. If you get it right, you might find this shorter-trouser look actually has a few advantages. Let me try to convince you.

First, the science. It all began with an American designer called Thom Browne who about 10 years ago decided to reinvent the proportion of men's tailoring. He designed his suits with sleeves that only reached down so far above the wrists, high waists that looked as if they were being hitched up by braces and trousers that finished well above the ankles. The overall look was as if you had either borrowed your little brother's suit for the day, or the dry cleaner owed you an apology.

I remember spotting a few gentlemen of fashion wearing these suits soon after they came out and there is no doubt it did look rather peculiar; there was something a little Charlie Chaplin or Buster Keaton about this almost comical silhouette. But, as is so often the case, the idea was soon emulated, toned down and before long didn't look so odd after all.

Men's fashion would never win an Olympic medal; it's the tortoise to womenswear's hare. It can take decades, sometimes even a century, for the way we dress to dramatically change. But Browne's idea reinvented the shape of our suits for the first time since the 1980s, and whether you're aware of it or not, any suit you buy today – from the high street or from Savile Row – will be under its influence. Jackets are now a tad more snug (excess snacks or not), sleeves are narrower and trousers no longer land on top of your shoe in a fug of folds. Most alteration tailors today will advise you to have the hem skimming the top of your shoe rather than smothering it.

There's method to all this madness. A slightly shorter trouser has a number of physical advantages: the shorter the trouser, the longer and leaner your leg looks; the less fabric there is dropping onto your shoe; the fewer unsightly folds and creases will develop farther up; and there's no doubt that the look lends the wearer a slightly more youthful, contemporary air.

But if the thought of hacking off the bottoms of your expensive suit trousers is an uncomfortable one, experiment instead with your off-duty ones. The easiest and more popular way to adopt this trend is with a pair of good old chinos – and you don't need to get them shortened. The most effective way is just to roll them up (never more than twice or you'll look like Janette Krankie). This will give you a casual, carefree look, especially if you team them with a pair of deck shoes or, if you want to be smarter, a tasselled loafer. Think Paul Newman or Jean-Paul Belmondo for inspiration.

If the weather's dodgy, wear them with a pair of regatta striped socks, but ideally you'll go socks free... and this is where the controversy kicks in. Men's feet do not generally get a good press, a fact not helped by the number of Hobbit-based films you can stream.

Unfortunately, men's ankles have been tarred with the same hairy brush as Tolkien's characters and some — mostly the opposite sex — claim that anything of ours below the waist should be hidden. Actually, our ankles are fine, and a touch of shin (ideally not too pasty) won't frighten the horses. And if they're hairy? Well, you're a bloke: they're supposed to be hairy. So ignore the doubters and you'll discover that if you roll up your chinos just a smidgen, feel the air on your ankles and the sole of your deck shoe underfoot, with a simple grey marled sweatshirt or T-shirt on top, the worries of the world will drop off your shoulders. You will instantly feel as if you're about to stroll along the Croisette in Cannes with Ali MacGraw, discuss Beat poetry with Allen Ginsberg, or head off on a road trip with Jack Kerouac. The strange thing about menswear is that every step forward takes you a few steps back. And we tend to find that a comfort.

Why you need to "outfit"

If you've watched *Downton Abbey*, or any drama set in the same era and class, you may have noticed how exhausting it was to spend the weekend with friends. Firstly, packing must have been a nightmare: selecting the right clothes to shoot in, lunch in, dine in, shag in, and faint in. In fact, getting packed and dressed for these weekends was so complex that no-one – male or female – was capable of doing it themselves. The ladies would have their maids help with hair and jewels and zips; the men would have valets to aid with cufflinks, bow ties and sliding into jackets.

Alan Hollinghurst's novel, *The Stranger's Child*, also dwells on the social pitfalls of staying in grand houses at the beginning of the last century – most of all, the unpleasant fact that you didn't get to unpack your own suitcase. You would see it taken up to your bedroom in the knowledge that a complete stranger would soon be rifling through your underwear.

Even today, these practices still exist in some of the country's grander houses. A friend of mine used to stay with the late Duke of Westminster and his family. The Grosvenors were, by all accounts, charming and hospitable, but he had to endure the stress of not only being dressed correctly at various times of the day, but also making sure he always had the right cash to tip the servants at the end of his stay.

Fortunately, most of us don't have to worry about such social conundrums today, but we are still likely to spend a few days with relatives or friends at some point each year. And if the stay coincides with a party, festive occasion or life event, then packing can potentially become cumbersome.

Like me, you probably loathe packing and leave it all to the last minute, and then bung a whole load of stuff into your bag hoping that 70% of it will be appropriate, 50% of it clean. Well, you need to approach things a little differently; you need to do something that is referred to in Fashionland as "outfitting". You can butch it up and call it something else if that helps, but outfitting is when you work out, and lay out, each outfit you're going to wear for every occasion you will face on your trip before packing it. Yes, it's like doing homework, but it's truly the best way to ensure that you have everything you need, that you don't overpack, and that, once you're there, you don't need to waste any time at all deciding what to wear.

A certain fashion editor, let's call him Gareth, that I used to work with would spend hours "outfitting" before he travelled to the biannual fashion shows in Milan and Paris. Last time I saw him, he had outfitted so obsessively the night before he flew out of London, laying each extravagant ensemble carefully out on his marital bed, that he failed to notice that it was 2am and his heavily pregnant wife was standing patiently by the door hoping to get a little shut-eye before their three-year-old woke.

Even if you're not heading off for the weekend, but just to the office or laptop the following morning, I'd still advise you to "outfit" the night before. Outfits chosen last thing at night (unless you're drunk) are usually more successful than those chosen first thing in the morning. Not only do you usually have more time at night, but the clothes-choosing section of your brain functions more effectively than it does shortly after you have just woken up from a deep sleep. At my age, your eyes work better, too. It takes a good 40 minutes before mine can focus properly each morning. It's an act of self-defence, of course. If I could actually see what I looked like first thing, I would never make it outside at all.

Nailing vacation wear

We're pretty confident on how to dress for an office – a good suit, crisp shirt, smart tie and polished shoes usually does the trick (for those who still go to offices) – but it's when we switch the Out Of Office sign on and head off for a vacation (for those who still have vacations) that we sometimes lose our way. Although men don't like being told what to do or how to dress, neither do we like getting things wrong. So I'd like you to think of the following as suggestions rather than rules on how to look good each summer.

T-shirts

The humble T-shirt should be a simple item to choose, and yet so many of us get it wrong. The following styles are best avoided:

1. Patterns. If you're over 30, avoid any brightly coloured, bold designs featuring flowers, animals or slogans. They are very fashionable and look great on teenagers on TikTok, but less appropriate on you on Facebook.

2. The black T-shirt is a perennial favourite with ageing rockers and reality TV stars who've spent too much time in LA. Avoid.

3. Gaping necklines. Many men choose T-shirts that have low slung, baggy necklines (see V-neck T-shirts above).

The safest, most stylish option is a classic white T-shirt. There is no need to choose anything else: look at how they worked for James Dean and Marlon Brando.

Shorts

The current trend for short shorts is best avoided: you don't want to look like Sacha Baron Cohen's Bruno. But don't go too long or baggy either, as this will be unflattering. A pair of shorts in a brushed cotton or linen is ideal (and a good place to try a splash of colour). Cargo shorts are popular but avoid too many pockets as they will make you look bulky. You don't want to be mistaken for a gap-year student.

Socks should never be worn with shorts. Fine for the cat-walk, not for the boardwalk.

Footwear

If you find sandals a bit scary, the safest and most stylish choices this summer are espadrilles, Do not consider Crocs or flip-flops.

Swimwear

Not everybody needs to know your religion, mole count or grooming habits from your choice of trunks: leave the Speedos for the gym bunnies on Mykonos. Neither, however, do you want to opt for long, baggy board shorts that will make you look like a wannabe Aussie surfer. Opt instead for a tailored pair of swim shorts that fall halfway down your thigh.

Polo shirts

These, an ubiquitous summer staple, can all too easily look bland, ill-fitting and ageing. To avoid looking too nerdy, choose a style that is tailored, slim-fitting and ideally in a pastel colour that you can team with a light-hued trouser. A loose design, worn with loose-fitting chinos, will make you look middle-aged. For inspiration look at old pictures of President Kennedy sailing around Hyannis Port.

Chinos

The perfect halfway-house trousers, since they can work on and off duty. Best in traditional khaki or navy (although red is popular), make sure that they're not too baggy or too long. A chino should finish at least half an inch above your shoe or trainer (ideally with a turn-up). At the weekend, they look best teamed with a white trainer or a deck shoe; for work they look good with a loafer or lightweight brogue (no socks required).

Don't wear your black suit belt with shorts or chinos. A woven leather-trimmed or canvas belt will look much more sprightly and appropriate.

Accessories

Coloured beaded or roped bracelets are popular with the jet-setters in Ibiza. These look best grouped together, rather than worn singularly.

On holiday, many of us end up carting all the stuff we

need for the beach in a bag that our partner has given us to carry. This is often not ideal; it might well be emblazoned with a big logo or a Hello Kitty! design. Come prepared with your own beach-ready carrier: choose something casual and unponcy – a simple blue canvas tote, for example.

Baseball caps are great if you're a paparazzi-avoiding celebrity, or Jay-Z, but otherwise best avoided if you're over 25. Old-fashioned bucket hats are back in fashion and have a certain quirky charm.

Avoid dark navy or black jeans and opt for a more washed denim in a looser fit. A pair of weathered jeans (but no rips; you're not Bros), rolled up once (or twice) at the ankle teamed with a white T-shirt and a pair of espadrilles is hard to beat. Denim jackets have also made a comeback. Again, opt for a washed finish and team with a T-shirt and a pair of cotton shorts or chinos. Do not do double denim.

A grey sweatshirt is perfect over a T-shirt. And, in a preppy way, worn over a white shirt and slim striped tie for smarter occasions.

There are so many styles of sunglass, it's hard to choose. Avoid big, coloured frames or blue mirrored lenses. A chic, safe option is a pair of dark lenses with a rounded tortoise-shell frame. Or Ray-Bans – they suit everyone.

Unless you have extraordinarily pumped guns or are in a boy band, short-sleeved shirts will make you look like an extra from *The Office*. Just roll up the sleeves of an ordinary shirt.

The best option for summer formality is a navy blazer

(soft and unstructured). You can slip one over a T-shirt or formal shirt, with smart trousers or chinos, with or without a tie, and it will look just right. A navy blazer is the most versatile item that you can buy.

Panama hats. Admittedly, they're a bit of a statement, but they can look rather dashing. You just have to look confident and make sure you don't resemble Mr Samgrass from *Brideshead Revisited*. Don't wear them on the back of your head.

Although most summer raincoats come in taupe, navy is much more versatile. Navy looks better worn over a light suit (you can have too many shades of beige). Plus, if you shove it into your briefcase, it won't show up the creases as much as a light mac.

You can always just watch it

Men are happy to talk about watches with each other. Watches are more machine than jewellery. Although the primary function of a watch – to tell the time – has been rendered pretty much obsolete by the invention of cell phones, the global luxury watch market is still worth around $7b. How come we are we still buying them? Why do heads of state still give watches to their hosts on the occasion of state visits? Why did Bernie Madoff own 17 Rolexes and seven Cartiers? It wasn't so long ago that your father would hand you a gold-plated watch on your 21st birthday and that would be that. It never crossed a man's mind that he might need to add another two or three by the time he hit 30. And it certainly never crossed his mind that when he reached 40 he might be grateful to receive a smart wooden box with different felt-lined compartments in which to keep his "collection" of watches.

Watches have stopped being merely timekeepers; they have become creations that showcase craftsmanship, tradition, technology and innovation. They've become a Savile Row suit, Mayfair member's club and Nasa spaceship rolled into one package that can sit neatly on your wrist.

The only other item that men comfortably use to express themselves, or to show off with, is their car. But the flashy car is becoming less popular: not only are cars big, expensive, environmentally unsound, dangerous and déclassé; they have another major disadvantage compared to the watch: they are parked in the garage rather than being displayed where all can see them. A watch is the Porsche you can wear on your wrist.

The technology used in today's watches – whether it's an Apple Watch or a Patek Philippe – is crucial. We men are, intrinsically, nerdy; we love nothing more than an item that not only looks good but has myriad functions and a construction that will have taken a lot of craftsmen a lot of time. One highly collectible Patek Philippe model, the limited-edition Calibre 89 – once the world's most complicated watch – has 33 functions (including telling you the time of sunrise and sunset, indicating leap years, providing the date of Easter, as well as a thermometer and a moon phase display) and 1,278 parts, which include 68 springs and 24 hands. One sold at auction in 2004 for more than $5m.

Whether a watch cost £50 or £5,000, we'll note what another bloke is sporting in the same way some women might take note of another's shoes. It's certainly harder to put a foot wrong with a watch purchase than it is with an item of clothing.

What to wear if you're marrying a man

Not so long ago, I got married to a bloke. There are two reasons why I still find this odd. One, because I'm a bloke, too (gay marriage was only made legal in the UK in 2014) and two, because last time I got married it was to a woman. If you're confused, imagine how I feel.

It's not just me who still finds same-sex matrimony per-plexing. When I visited the local town hall to register our intent to marry (my partner had to go on a different day due to work schedules), the sweet, elderly registrar welcomed me into her office and we sat down to fill in the forms.

"Have you ever changed your name?" she asked.

"Well, yes, as it happens," I replied. (When my mother remarried, which was often, she would sometimes have our names changed by deed poll so they matched hers.)

"Oh," said the registrar. "Do you have the change of name deeds with you?"

"Yes," I replied. "Here you go."

She carried on typing, slowly.

"This is obviously your first marriage?" she asked, moments later.

"Actually, no. I was married before. To a lady."

"Oh," she said, surprised again. "Do you have your divorce papers?"

I handed them over.

"Oh," she said again. "You were married to that opinionated lady from *The Sunday Times*."

Yes, I was. We ploughed through some of the other questions.

"Will either of you be having best men?" she asked.

"No, we're keeping numbers very small – immediate family only."

"Hmmm," she nodded. "Will either of you be given away by a parent?

I snorted. "Err, no, no."

"Hmmm, who will hand you the rings when it comes to that part of the service?" she asked.

"Oh, umm, I'll probably get one of my kids to do that."

There was a long pause.

"Oh, I see," she said. "How nice."

Booking a three-day honeymoon was no less complicated. I emailed the hotel – a small, family-run one in the South of France that only takes reservations by email – asking if they had a quality room available. Thankfully, they did. I wrote and asked if I could see a picture of the one that was free to placate my control-freak concerns.

"Unfortunately we don't have pictures we can send," she emailed back.

Fair enough, I replied, explaining that I only wanted to be sure because it would be my honeymoon.

"No problem, monsieur," she wrote. "We will make sure you and your wife have a lovely room."

Aah. I worried that if I didn't correct her, there might be some confusion on our arrival and so decided I'd better explain the situation.

Actually it will be me and my husband, I wrote back, adding a wink emoji in the hope that she would see I understood that these things aren't as clear-cut as they used to be.

"Ha," she replied. "Many apologies. I assumed you were a man because it said Jeremy at the bottom of the email.

At this point, I gave up. I would have to risk puzzled looks at check-in.

The reason I've told you this is that sometimes the dilemmas facing same-sex marriage, all these years later, extend to what two grooms should wear on their wedding day. A big frothy dress is usually out of the question – but not always (and each to their own) – but neither do you, I believe, want his'n'his matching suits. I've been to a few same-sex weddings and am always a little puzzled as to why grooms choose to wear the same outfits. It's disturbing enough when couples start to emulate each other's mannerisms, and finish each other's sentences, let alone dress all matchy-matchy.

The trick is to look as if you're getting hitched to each other, with equal excitement and respect, but not to look as if you're both on the way to the same board meeting. We opted for two off-the-peg suits that I then got tailored to an even better fit. One of us wore a grey suit; the other a navy one, and we both wore ties and buttonholes of a similar design but different colourway. I think it worked well. But ultimately your wedding – same sex or not – is your wedding. And that means you can both wear exactly what you want. Invite who you want. And drink as much as you want. Who cares what the rest of us think.

Are you ever too old for fashion?

Are you old? Perhaps you're not sure. After all, it's hard to tell these days. Whether you're 25 or 55, the chances are you wear the same clothes, frequent a gym, party a little too hard on occasion and think a lot about work.

Because most of us eat well, exercise, moisturise and keep our hair in shape (above and below the waistline), we look younger for longer. And if we're lucky, we feel fitter, too, thanks to statins, juicers and fitness apps. Your age is no longer the number of years you've been alive, you tell yourself; it's the number of years you feel (or can get away with posting on your Tinder/Grindr profile).

Is this good news? Mostly, yes. As long as you really are as fit as you feel. But you have to be self-aware: aware that however many wrinkles you've zapped with the Botox needle, your coronary arteries still know the date written on your birth certificate; aware that you don't want to be grandpa disco at the party (never be the last to leave); aware that hangovers take longer to repair; and aware that if you're over

45 and you fall over, it's no longer called "a fall" – it's called "having a fall" and it hurts.

A few years ago, a survey by researchers at University College, London, revealed that older-feeling adults were about 40% more likely to die than younger-feeling adults of the same age. So if you feel younger than your age, you'll live longer. Hoorah: the key to living longer is self-delusion. Easy.

Of course, we've tried to give a name to this "younger for longer" generation: middle youth is the most frequently used, and it's only a matter of time before they're called YoLos. But really, there's long been an appropriate name for it: middle age. It's just that middle age is more all-encompassing than it used to be: it's drainpipe jeans and sneakers as well as pipes and slippers. Both qualify. You can be young with an old heart: think Manny in *Modern Family* or Andy Barbour in *The Goldfinch*; or older with a young heart: think Keith Richards or Captain Tom Moore.

The reality is that the YoLo (told you it was only a matter of time) has the best of both worlds: he still looks good, and yet knows more and cares less (what others think). The two Cs (entwined like a Chanel logo) that you greet with joy as you journey into middle age are Confidence (whatevs) and Consequence (told you). Annoying for others, admittedly, but so heavenly to so often say exactly what you think and nearly always be right.

The reason I mention all this is that the menswear world seems rather fond of its elders at the moment. Street-style blogs savour snappy middle-aged dressers such as Robert Rabensteiner of L'Uomo Vogue and menswear-retailer-turned-designer Nick Wooster; many of the ad campaigns at the moment feature handsome, grey-haired old-timers such as John Pearson or Aiden Shaw; five years ago Selfridge's even swapped its annual Bright Young Things campaign for one called Bright Old Things, where a number of artists, designers and musicians in their late forties to mid-eighties were given their own windows to design and their own space to sell their products in-store. Selfridges, explaining the campaign, said that "old is as subjective as it is irrelevant". The fashion world has (maybe out of necessity rather than kindness) embraced all ages. There's something for everyone.

I was having a drink with a handful of friends in someone's London flat, pre-Covid, one Tuesday evening, when Lindsay Lohan turned up fresh from the theatre. Even though I knew the evening had the possibility to be a fun one, it was a school night and so I sensibly left at 11.30pm. "I'm sorry to be so rude and leave almost as soon as you get here," I said to the actress as I made my way to the door. "It's not rude," replied Lohan, puffing on a cigarette at the window, "just boring." LiLo put this YoLo right in his place.

Sartorial tips for the over fifties

Trousers

The most popular trend for trousers, and one that looks as if it will continue for quite some time, is trousers with a

VAIN GLORIOUS

drawstring or elasticated waist. Who would have thought? These are not only cake-friendly; there is also no need to find your glasses before trying to do up the fiddly clasp or button fly. Don't use elasticated waists as a gateway into tracksuits, though. While some of you may be able to get away with a pair of grey sweatpants outside the gym (but not outside the home), worn with a matching tracksuit top you veer into questionable territory.

Trouser length

Make sure your trousers don't fold heavily onto your shoes like Simon Cowell's (he wears his like that to disguise his Cuban heels). A slightly shorter trouser length will make you look taller.

Finding the right fit

There are a few simple things you can do to update your wardrobe that will make it seem fresher and smarter (and I don't mean a trip to the dry cleaner's). Clothes that fit properly will always make you look slimmer and younger, so anything that's too loose, too long or too sloppy you should get tightened up by a tailor. It will give old pieces, including you, a new lease of life.

Good impression

And there is nothing more youthful than a well-pressed white shirt – keep the wrinkles on your face, but off your clothes.

136

Cufflinks and short-sleeved shirts

Don't ask me why, but cufflinks and short-sleeved polo shirts are ageing. Try to avoid them.

Old friends

The chances are there are a few items buried in the back of your wardrobe that have come back into fashion: corduroys and blousons are in favour again this winter, for example. If you still own either of these items, leave the jumbo-cord ones there because they are unlikely to be flattering, and call your blouson a bomber jacket. No-one says blouson any more.

Colours

As mentioned earlier, navy is far more flattering as you get older. And being a little older doesn't preclude you from wearing strong colours, as long as you stick with just one – on a shirt, tie, sweater or pocket square, for example. Mix too many colours and you might look as if you've just been voted off *Strictly Come Dancing*.

Sneakers

I moved into a new house recently and, as I unpacked my boxes of shoes – some of which had been in storage for years – and laid them all out on the floor in order of purchase, I could see my adult years told through a series of soles. It was like the ascent of man illustrated with leather uppers. I noticed, too, that the number of trainers I owned had diminished as the years went by. As I entered middle age, I'd obviously deemed them inappropriate.

As you get older, choosing a pair of trainers is not a task you can undertake lightly. Invest in the wrong ones and you'll look more ASBO than *à la mode*. And, as you head into your forties, you also don't want to discover you're sporting the same hi-tops as Justin Bieber. In fact, if you're in your forties, you shouldn't be wearing hi-tops at all.

This is the problem with middle-aged trainers (or sneakers if you're living in the States or under 40): the sartorial pitfalls are myriad. Many, more sensible men ditch them altogether once they've hit 39; after all, a scuffed-up pair of brown leather brogues or loafers is always going to look more stylish and age-appropriate. But there is something about a sneaker that is hard to resist. Without wishing to put too much philosophy behind a pair of soft, leather lace-ups, a sneaker conveys a sense of energy, or activity; something that appeals as you approach middle age. Even though it's more about aesthetics than athletics, it demonstrates a certain vigour.

Vigour or not, I stopped wearing sneakers about six years ago. I no longer felt it necessary to waste time worrying whether you're meant to thread the laces of your sneakers all the way to the top, have the tongue hanging in or outside the fastening, tuck your jeans into the hi-top, leave them looking box-fresh or let them get a tad grimy. Nor did I find it comforting to discover my teenage kids vying for the same footwear as me: "All right, Pops. Dope Nikes!"

But then, a couple of years ago, a number of brands started producing slick, smart versions that appeared urbane and understated; designs that added just the right degree of sporty sophistication to take the stuffiness out of an otherwise conventional office ensemble: soft, brown leather or suede sneakers with patent toe caps and elegant white rubber soles that barely smacked of sportswear at all. Comfortingly, these were far more Pop's than hip-hop's.

Of course, not every middle-aged sneaker-wearer is a fan of this luxury lace-up combo. There is a rival faction – and I'm sure you've got friends in this group – who remain obsessively loyal to the retro sneaker; the footwear of their youth. Current favourite with the retro-sneaker-heads is the Nike Air Jordan 6 in VI Retro black or white Infrared. The Jordan sub-brand of Nike is revered the world over and arguably the cause of the entire sneaker-freaker phenomenon in the first place. Otherwise, for the man who wants to pretend he was a skateboard fanatic in his youth, Vans is having a huge resurgence at the moment, with the classic Old Skool leading the way.

The third element in the should-you-or-shouldn't-you footwear conundrum is the statement sneaker, popular with most of the big design houses. These chunky, elaborate designs have cruelly been nicknamed "dad sneakers" by the fashion fraternity. This doesn't mean they should be worn by dads. Fortunately, most of these age-inappropriate trainers have such long names that anyone over the age of 50 is unlikely to remember what they're called – so avoid putting a pair of Nike + Acronym Air VaporMax Flyknit Moc 2s on your wishlist.

Safer and chicer is a pair of simple white trainers that can look smart and modern when worn with trousers or chinos, or even with a suit; a look favoured by Sir Paul McCartney. Or a pair of white Jack Purcells: they're plain, inexpensive and have been worn by everyone from James Dean to Steve McQueen. And somehow, you can't get more age appropriate than McQueen.

The perils of dressing bravely

A few years ago, when I was a rookie magazine editor, our team would have to spend weeks on end, twice a year, visiting designers' showrooms and looking at their latest creations. Much of what they displayed was, of course, delightful, and we would coo and praise accordingly. But there were always a small handful of labels – it would be mean to name and shame them here – whose success we found unfathomable. An enthusiastic public relations assistant would show us the latest collection, and we'd be lost for words. Who on earth could create a pair of shoes like those and think that they were either lovely or wearable? We would try to hide our sniggers and conjure up a compliment that didn't sound too insincere.

After years of practice, we came up with two that fitted the bill. The adjective we used most often, which usually left the PR thinking we'd liked what we'd seen, was "very brave".

As we stared in awe at a shoe made from multicoloured croc-odile skins, embossed with gold snakes and topped off with oversized white leather tassels, the words "very brave" seemed fitting. The other phrase, more appropriate when confronted with the creator of the controversial item, was: "Wow, the collection was just… so… so you." If paired with a warm smile and a firm handshake, the designer usually looked pleased to hear this.

Fashion compliments don't always travel well, though. What makes sense in the UK doesn't always translate so well in Italy. A former colleague of mine, after watching a show by a big Italian label featuring lots of Aran knits, flow-ing tweed coats and chunky shoes, kissed the designer on both cheeks and cheerfully told him the collection was "very Midsomer Murders". When she tried to explain what the show was about, the designer looked a little puzzled. "Can you please send me the DVDs?" he asked. "We must watch these." Weeks of angst followed as she wondered what the big fashion house made of the boxset she'd sent of DCI Tom Barnaby solving endless mysteries involving old ladies found dead at the bottom of their timber-framed staircases.

I mention this because the word "brave" can be, as dem-onstrated above, a double-edged sword. Brave, when it comes to clothes, can be something quite admirable; but it can also be something wholly awful. There's a fine line, for example, between someone dressing like a dandy or dressing like a dick. While perusing a book of photographs by the art-ist Peter Schlesinger – a former lover of David Hockney who photographed the bohemian arty party set of the 60s and 70s – I was struck by a picture he'd taken in 1970 of Hockney sitting with Cecil Beaton in the latter's Wiltshire conservatory. Hockney is seated in a wicker chair with his signature mop of peroxide hair and oversized round spectacles, wearing a pastel-pink tweed suit with a big baby-blue-and-brown windowpane check, a brown silk tie with large pink spots and one brick-red sock and one emerald-green sock. Beaton, meanwhile, is clad in a moss-green corduroy suit with a knitted waistcoat teamed with an extravagantly tied lime-green silk cravat and matching socks, all finished off with a large-rimmed brown fedora. How marvellous they both look, I thought. Yet imagine the comments even from my friends if I wore either of those outfits today. In fact, imagine the sarcastic comments if I only adopted the mismatched socks. Everyone would just put it down to early-onset Alzheimer's.

I suppose what makes brave commendable with dressing is when it feels genuine rather than contrived; when it's part of the personality rather than instead of a personality; when it's a symptom rather than the cause. Hockney's love of colour, shape and convention-breaking is represented in his work, love life and – last and least – his wardrobe. Despite his arresting attire, when Hockney walks into a room it is his success as an artist not the colour of his socks that strikes you first.

Hilton Als writes in the foreword to Schlesinger's book that the world was a much more open place when his photographs were taken than it is today. You didn't need to be so brave back in 1970 to nip out for a pint of milk in an array of mismatched rainbow hues. But I think the world has changed once more since that book was published. I think the world is, largely, more open once more. Up to a point. If you look a little too contrived, you still might find one of the *Esquire* team coming over and telling you how brave you look.

Chapter 7

Sit Back and Exercise

THERE WAS AN ARTICLE, PUBLISHED IN the Canadian magazine, *Macleans*, way back in 1959, titled: "Can you loaf your way to a better figure?" Its focus was a number of machines that had been invented that claimed to do your exercise for you. These contraptions enabled you to curl up on the sofa and plug yourself into the electronic equivalent of four hours of sit-ups, lie on a rocking couch and treat your body to the equivalent of 36 holes of golf, or lay back on your bed, light a fag and put your muscles through a virtual 10-mile walk.

Although the Relax-A-Cizor comes a close second, my favourite of these inventions is the Stauffer Office Gym. This relic of the 1950s looks like a smart foldaway bed (as if designed by the architect and furniture wizard Eileen Gray), but has a motorised cushion that sits under your hips and rocks your pelvis (or other parts of the body, if required) at a speed of around 120 times a minute. The sub-*Madmen* launch ad for it has a slightly podgy male executive, dressed in traditional work attire (but without the jacket) lying back and smiling at the camera while his slim, chirpy secretary sits happily on the chair beside him taking down dictation. The copy states: "If your doctor says you must reduce without strain, here's how to lose that old-fashioned bay window... The Stauffer Office Gym is motorised to do your exercise for you by gently rhythmic motion. No discomfort."

If only it were true. The *Macleans* article features testimonials from numerous customers who claim the various inventions work, but the medical experts quoted are unimpressed. Disappointingly, they claim that according to medical theory, "improvements in muscle performance result from a sophistication of the brain; they neither begin nor end in any change in the inert red meat, called muscle, that the brain governs". Humbugs.

The mainstream fitness craze for men first truly kicked in halfway through the last century when American life insurance companies started warning a generation of overweight executive-level middle-aged workers with high stress levels and sedentary lifestyles that they were heading for an early grave. In 1953, according to Lynne Luciano's revealing book, *Looking Good: Male Body Image in Modern America* (Hill and Wang, 2000), *Time* magazine announced that "America was becoming a nation of fat people". Employers started to encourage workers to eat healthier and exercise more, and women were proffered advice on "the care and feeding of business executives" or even "how to keep a husband alive". The beer belly was described as "the kiss of death to any man who seriously wants to get ahead in his career".

Today it feels as if we might have come full circle. By 2030, an estimated 20% of the world's population will be obese. And, once again, it's the middle-ranking executive who is most at risk. According to a report in 2020 by the Centers for Disease Control and Prevention in the States, obesity rates for men are highest for middle-income groups.

Over the last 60 years, in particular, the way we men have wanted, or been told, our bodies should look has varied in size and structure dramatically. And the way we've tried to achieve those goals along the way has been equally contrary.

After the initial physical fitness regimes that began in the 1950s, championed by US presidents such as Eisenhower and Kennedy, the 1960s saw a temporary softening when clothes became more important than the bodies beneath them. The 1970s changed all that with the rise of youth culture and the fashion for aerobics classes, health clubs and then, towards the end of the decade, the cult of the bodybuilder: in 1977, after Arnold Schwarzenegger had won six Mr Olympia competitions, a documentary about his success on the bodybuilding circuit, *Pumping Iron*, was released, and it made him a star. He and his physique went on to become a Hollywood icon, to marry a Kennedy and become a governor of California.

As Schwarzenegger's profile grew, so did everyone's muscles. In the 1980s, bodies got bigger and gym clothes smaller.

You wore your health on your sleeve-less T. Looking fit was the sign of a high achiever: it meant a better job and a better sex life. So much so that in the 1990s gyms even started to look like nightclubs. The New York gym impresario, David Barton, led the way by introducing low lighting, thumping live DJ sets and peacock-friendly changing rooms into his Manhattan fitness temples. Barton's famously showy mantras included: "No pecs, no sex" and "Look better naked."

Over the last 20 years, approaches to fitness have become, like everything else, more diverse: as well as the gym bunnies pumping iron and downing foul-smelling protein shakes, there are the runners zipping past us on pavements as they breathe in the traffic fumes and splutter Covid over everyone, there are the salubrious studios filled with yummy mummies with muscle groups toned by years of yoga, pilates and Ottolenghi lemon and fregola salads. And there are the men, like me, with dad bods, who, instead of going to the gym, go onto ebay and see if they can score a vintage Relax-A-Cizor (you can and they're less than $60) or a Stauffer Office Gym (no luck so far).

Even today, after so much progress in gender equality, there is still an extraordinarily unfair chasm between what men and women can expect to get away with regarding how society judges their bodies. When Germaine Greer first published *The Female Eunuch* in 1970, she commented: "Is it too much to ask that women be spared the daily struggle for superhuman beauty in order to offer it to the caresses of a subhumanly ugly mate?" She had a point. And it still resonates today. The author Caitlin Moran recently moaned in *The Times* (August 2020) about how unfair it was that dad bods were deemed attractive by women and not the other way around.

The phrase "dad bod" was coined in a blog by a 19-year-old American law student called Mackenzie Pearson. She wrote: "The dad bod is a nice balance between a beer gut and working out. The dad bod says, 'I go to the gym occasionally – but I also drink heavily on the weekends and enjoy eating eight slices of pizza at a time.' It's not an overweight guy, but it isn't one with washboard abs, either. There is just something about the dad bod that makes boys seem more human, natural and attractive."

Indeed, research conducted by the US gym chain Planet Fitness in 2019 found that, of its mixed-sex clients, 46% said that a dad bod made them feel relaxed, and 78% said a dad bod represented a man who was comfortable in his own skin.

While for many men a dad bod is worn as a badge of honour, for others it's a big problem. Body image pressure is one of the strongest instigators for eating disorders in men. Scroll through Instagram and you'll see millions of men of all ages showing off the desired body of the moment: lean with hard, toned muscle. They look like a pack of waxed Wolverines. Whatever your age, that body isn't an easy one to emulate.

The National Eating Disorders Association says that many men have misconceived notions about their weight and physique, particularly the potency of muscularity. "Most males would like to be lean and muscular, which typically represents the 'ideal' male body type," it reports. "Muscle dysmorphia, a subtype of body dysmorphic disorder, is an emerging condition that primarily affects male bodybuilders. Compulsions include spending many hours in the gym, squandering excessive amounts of money on supplements, abnormal eating patterns, or use of steroids." Today, one in three people suffering from an eating disorder is male.

Liposuction continues to be one of the most popular elective cosmetic surgeries chosen by men, as it has been for decades, despite the fact it's a seriously invasive procedure, doesn't deal with the root cause of the problem, rarely has long-lasting results and, for God's sake, killed Kanye West's mum.

So on the one hand, we have a rise in male bulimia, body dysmorphic disorder and exercise addiction (exercise releases endorphins and dopamine, the same neurotransmitters released during drug use). On the other, we have a problem with obesity. The danger with the latter was highlighted once more with the outbreak of Covid-19. Being overweight put you at greater risk of serious illness or death from the virus. According to UK government statistics, nearly 8% of critically ill patients with Covid-19 in intensive care units, including the prime minister, Boris Johnson, were morbidly obese (a Body Mass Index of 40 or more). The government subsequently introduced its Better Health campaign banning TV advertising before 9pm for foods high in fat, salt and sugar and "buy one get one free" snack promotions, ordering calorie counts to be placed on menus, and urging everyone to get active and eat better.

Obviously, it's the get-active-and-eat-better approach we should pay the most attention to. And thankfully, the government isn't the only institution promoting this. Healthy eating and regular cardio exercise – as exemplified during lockdown by fitness and diet coaches such as Joe Wicks hosting workouts on their YouTube channels – are catching on. We learned that we can now lose weight by watching telly. What's not to like?

I've tried personal trainers (they talk too much and make you eat too little); healthy meal boxes delivered daily to your home (too expensive and they were frequently nicked before I'd collected them from the doorstep); and the blood analysis diet (you send off a blood sample and they tell you what food types you can eat. Mine came back saying avoid everything but air). I have even done 10 days at a fasting clinic in Germany (they should call it a farting clinic since you ate nothing but cabbage soup). I have, however, found two treatments available today that are not a million miles away from the ones featured in that 1959 article; ones that potentially do enable you to "loaf your way to a better figure".

One is a treatment called CoolSculpting. It's a quick-fix – no surgery, no downtime – procedure that freezes the fat cells in the part of your body being treated. Once frozen, they crystallise and die before being excreted via your body's lymphatic system (this takes between four and six months, boringly, but at least they are gone for good). The attractive part of this treatment is that all you have to do is lie on a couch while the device – which looks a bit like an iron – is placed on your body and freezes the selected area of tissue. I chose to lose two small areas of stubborn fat from my lower back. Initially it's a bit uncomfortable, as if someone has placed a couple of packs of frozen peas on there, but you soon get used to it. After 30 minutes, I got dressed and returned to work. My back did feel a little numb for a few days after, but nothing more ominous (cold doesn't damage other cells in the way it does fat cells, so there is little chance of damage to the skin or tissue). Research published in *Medical News Today* and elsewhere suggests CoolSculpting does actually work to remove small areas of fat. Four months later, I studied the before and after pictures and the fat had indeed disappeared from my lower back to leave a more streamlined silhouette.

If CoolSculpting can help to get rid of unwanted fat, whether it's on your bum or stomach, how about a bit of muscle definition, too? Well today's Relax-A-Cizor is called EMsculpt. This contraption uses "high-intensity electro-magnetic technology that induces rapid and deep muscle contractions", which apparently force your muscle tissue to rebuild, lift and firm. Once again, you simply lie on a couch – hooray! – and the device is placed on the area being treated: in my case on my abdomen. This treatment needs a course of about four sessions of 30 minutes, ideally over a period of two to three days. It does feel peculiar as your muscles endure a super-intense workout while you lie there doing nothing – as though an alien was doing 20,000 sit-ups for you – but according to the studies done on the procedure, it creates about 16% muscle development in the area treated.

Six weeks later, I was convinced the muscle definition on my stomach appeared more visible than before. Was it wishful thinking? Was my mirror telling fibs again? Even if this was the case, apparently the psychological and physical benefit of taking a decision to lose weight or improve your body can be a good first step. As one of the doctors quoted in *Macleans* magazine says: "It's the power of positive thinking." Think yourself thin. I think someone's written that book already.

The truth is that even if I did get a better-looking body from these treatments, it doesn't mean I got a healthier one. As my doctor unkindly pointed out at my last annual health check, while my weight may have stayed the same for the last few years, and my body is in relatively good shape for my age: "Remember, Jeremy, you're still 55 on the inside and nothing can change that." Oh.

You can always distract with a tat

Friends are often surprised when they spot that I have three tattoos. I'm often surprised, too, since I forget that I have them myself until they peer out from under the sleeves of my T-shirt for three days each summer. My mum is horrified by them. She always asks, as do other critics, what happens when I get old: who wants to look at tattoos on wrinkly arms?

There are two answers to that. One is that nobody looks at your naked limbs when you're old, tattoo or not, so it's probably the best time to have one if you're a tad self-conscious.

The second is that if you do have to take your clothes off in public, you might be grateful that eyes will be drawn first to the tattoos you're sporting rather than any other areas of your body. The chances are that the inkings will have fared better than the rest of you.

My first tattoo, which I got aged 32, was born from pure boredom. A few friends and I had rented a cottage in a small coastal town in Sussex for a summer weekend and I'd gone there a day early for some peace and quiet before the others arrived. Typically, it was pouring with rain, and after a few hours sheltering in the house, I decided to potter around the deserted town. There was nothing to peruse but shops selling plastic buckets and spades, sweet stores selling unappetising sticks of candy and a cinema that had recently closed down. Eventually, I stumbled across a dingy-looking tattoo parlour. Oh well, I thought, it might take up some of the afternoon.

I quickly chose an image of a gecko to be inked on one of my shoulder blades – a girl I had fancied at college had had one – and off we went. It was agony. Tattooing bony areas of the body is quite painful, and I was there for nearly two hours. When my friends arrived that evening, they couldn't believe there was a small lizard, covered in clingfilm, perched on my back. I was a little surprised, too. I didn't look like the sort of person who would have a tattoo, especially back then, in the pre-*Love Island* days, when a tramp stamp was a relative rarity. But since it was hidden away on the back of my shoulder, holidays aside, neither I nor anyone else saw it very often. My gecko didn't loom large in my life.

Ten years later, however, I began to yearn for a second tattoo, this time a larger, more colourful one on the top of my arm. It features a heart with an arrow in it, framed by a twisted rope and anchor. I hope it had nothing to do with the Jean-Paul Gaultier Le Male perfume ad, created by Pierre et Gilles, which featured a stylised Jean Genet-inspired sailor, but I suspect that subconsciously it did. I couldn't help but be amused by the incongruity of it being attached to me, my being more John Craven than Jean Genet in appearance.

The tattoo, which was done at the Family Business, a well-known tattoo parlour in east London, got quite good reviews. My friends looked to heaven but secretly liked it, and my ex-wife and teenage sons were seemingly impressed. A few years later, when my eldest son turned 18, he asked for a tattoo for his birthday. My youngest son did, too, when he reached the same age. It looked like the family from *Here Comes Honey Boo Boo* had moved into Primrose Hill.

Fast-forward one more decade, and the itch for ink returned once more. On my 52nd birthday, my husband gave me a gift voucher for a tattoo by Mo Coppoletta. Coppoletta owns the Family Business, gets booked up months and months in advance and has collaborated on projects with brands such as Rolls-Royce, Turnbull & Asser and Montblanc.

Coppoletta is the expert, so I asked him what he thought I should have done. I returned a week later to discover he had designed a large, intricate tattoo featuring a fierce-looking tiger pouncing from a fire-strewn sabre. It was extraordinary.

He suggested I had it tattooed on the upper half of the arm not already decorated by his colleague's heart and anchor. "Go for it," I said as breezily as I had to the man in the seaside town 20 years before.

Coppoletta began by testing different-sized cut-outs of the design to see what would suit the image and my arm the best. To be honest, I had so many emails to attend to on my phone I didn't pay much attention at this stage. It was the easiest way to avoid the endless buzz and prick of the minuscule needles jabbing in and out of my skin. After a couple of hours, as the pain began to build up – you can only block it out for so long – I peered down to see how it was looking. My eyes nearly popped out of my head, resembling those of the tiger that had just been inked onto my upper arm. The tattoo was enormous. Splendid, but enormous. It was practically a sleeve. Unlike the other one, it wouldn't disappear under a T-shirt. This one would be peering out at the world for most of the summer. Grrr!

That first session took four hours. It hurt. A fortnight later, I returned for another two-hour session to finish it off. A week later, the scabs were cleanly healed – a lot of nappy ointment on the scabbing is the trick – and my new tattoo was now ready to greet the world. Like me, many of my friends and colleagues (although the latter were too polite to say so) were quite alarmed by its size and vibrancy. A handful didn't believe it was real. There were the inevitable jokes, too. "The sabre handle looks like a giant tiger penis." "Who knew you were such a Kellogg's Frosties fan?"

"I didn't know Gucci sold stick-on tattoos." Ho, ho, ho.

This past summer, with no office to dress up for, my giant tiger tat has been out and about a great deal, brazenly creeping out from under every short-sleeved shirt I wear. As well as enjoying the age-inappropriate friendship my upper arm now has with this snarling Technicolor beast, I frequently look down and admire its beauty, admire the fact that someone was able to draw and colour such an accurate and intricate design onto a limb rather than a canvas and that, unlike the other paintings I've collected over the years, I get to take this one with me wherever I go.

And when one day, as gravity plays its usual cruel tricks, the tiger no longer clings quite as tightly to my upper arm as it does now, who cares? I've often thought about having a tattoo on my forearm; I may well end up with one there for free.

Conclusion

SURELY THERE ISN'T A MAN OR woman who doesn't look in the mirror and wonder who they are and who they're going to be. But does that make you vain?

According to the Collins English dictionary, a vain person is one who takes "an extreme pride in their own beauty, intelligence, or other good qualities".

In Greek mythology, the handsome Narcissus (from whom sprang the adjective narcissistic) was punished not for being obsessed with how he looked, but for treating those who fell in love with him, especially the nymph Echo and, in some translations of the myth, a young man called Ameinias, with callous disregard. In retribution, the gods made him fall in love with his own reflection in a pool of water. Unable to draw himself away from his mirror image, which of course he was physically unable to caress or kiss, he eventually died of thirst.

It's highly unlikely, however many treatments I try, that I will ever fall in love with my own reflection. After all these years, I think my reflection and I know each other too well to fall in love; we've reached the let's-just-be-friends stage. In fact, we're not really even that close; it's a very one-way relationship. "Mirror mirror on the wall, who's the fairest of them all?" No reply. Awks.

What's hard to remember is the age we are when we first look in a mirror and become aware of how we appear to others. That "Oh, I see. That's me." moment. After that realisation, our reflections become an external rather than an internal story – a mirror reveals how the outside world sees us rather than who we think we are inside. For those who are more insecure about their place in the world and where they fit in it, looking in the mirror becomes like a game of Chatroulette. What will I see today? Will I keep looking, or should I spin the wheel and hope that someone I like more stares back at me the next time? Some of us keep the wheel spinning for the rest of our lives, as well as placing bets on other tables, in the hope that, one day, we'll hit the jackpot.

In my early thirties, I became quite simply addicted to mirrors. And I'm not being flippant. If I didn't have access to a mirror, I would feel uneasy, distracted; instead of focusing on the conversation I was having, or the work I was doing, I would be fixating on when I could next check myself in a mirror. Like a heroin addict, I was worried about getting my next fix. And, believe me, this wasn't vanity in the Collins dictionary sense. I didn't look in the mirror, inhale my good looks and return to my desk or the dinner table on a self-satisfied high. I would look in the mirror, check whether anything "terrible" had happened to my face – lettuce in my teeth, or a bogey in my nose, for example – and then return to what I was doing, relaxed and happy in the knowledge that it was still the same as it was the last time I had checked. I was still in control of how I appeared to others.

This wasn't easy. I have worked in some big offices, which often means a long walk to the bathroom to check the mirrors. If there's someone else standing at the washbasins, that means you can't check your reflection quite as thoroughly as you would like to. The same with restaurants. If after eating the spinach that was served with your main course you want to check whether any of it ended up stuck between your teeth, it's quite a rigmarole to excuse yourself from the table, head to the restaurant's bathrooms and look in the mirror; again, ideally, without any other diners in there at the same time who might make you feel the need to hurry. When eating out, unless it's with friends or colleagues I know well, I will avoid ordering green vegetables, salads, or anything with coriander, that might get stuck in my teeth, despite loving the taste of all of them. Sometimes, if I imagine something is wedged in between my front teeth, and I can't go to check, I will talk for the rest of the meal through tight lips, cover my mouth when I laugh, even try and hurry the meal to an end. I can't focus on the occasion if, in my mind, there's the slightest possibility I might have teeth stuff. I even abbreviated teeth stuff to TS to use as a code with my wife, and then later with my husband, for when we were out for dinner. When the conversation was flowing, and our fellow diners were distracted, I would whisper across the table, "TS?", and pull an exaggerated smile so that they could clearly see my teeth. They would usually, perhaps always, nod that it was fine. I could then relax and continue to enjoy the evening. This phobia became so debilitating and time-consuming that I had to come up with shortcuts. When I was working at *The Sunday Times*, where my desk and computer faced a wall, I had small wing mirrors attached to each side of my computer. I joked to colleagues that this eccentricity was so that I could tell whether the newspaper's editor was coming up behind me (which the mirrors were actually useful for) but in fact it was so that I could regularly check my reflection without having to leave the desk. I was fully aware that there was very little damage that could happen to my face – there wasn't spinach flying through the air-conditioning units in the *Sunday Times* offices – but reason and rationality made no dent on my concerns. After *The Sunday Times*, when I became the editor of a magazine, I didn't feel the wing mirrors gave quite the right impression to my team and so went instead for small compact mirrors that could sit, less obtrusively, on the desk beside me. I shopped around and was able to find little leather-bound ones that, when face down, looked as if they were drinks mats, so nobody would know the truth. As the years went by, the addiction didn't subside, but technology made handling it a lot easier. Initially, I would rely on the camera on my iPhone. Press the reverse button and there is your reflection ready for a selfie. Any sign of something in my teeth, a spot on my forehead, snot in my nose? No, good, let's get back to the conversation. I never travel without a supply of floss picks either. The drawers in my desk at work are stacked high with them, my work bag is filled with them; they're scattered across the bottoms of suitcases, along the tops of bedside tables, by bathroom sinks; I even have to check all the pockets of my trousers before putting them in the wash for those familiar green or white plastic picks. They aren't good for the environment; nor, I suspect, with the frequency I use them, are they good for my teeth. Salvation eventually arrived in the form of a phone app called Mirror, which allows you to magnify your reflection. This has enabled me, when the urge to check my reflection hits me at inopportune moments, to pretend I'm checking an important text message. The odd faces I pull when reading "my text messages" – the ones needed to check my teeth and nostrils – I can explain away as shortsightedness. A therapist will sensibly tell you, as mine did, that when you can't control the chaos around you as a young child, you grow up determined to ensure that loss of control doesn't happen again. This can mean developing certain obsessive compulsive disorders, like the mirror one above, or an exhausting quest for perfection in your career, home and children. Happy face = happy life.

A hectic and emotionally disruptive childhood – my mother married four rather peculiar men in quick succession (one ran away, one was carted away, one passed away and the other we just told to piss off) – forced me, at a young age, into the role of peacemaker. My fall-back position: let's pretend everything's alright. So, quick, tidy the sitting room, put on a fresh shirt, comb your hair, put the kettle on. There now, see, everything is fine... Ooops, Daddy died. Well, never mind. At least he didn't make a mess. Tea's ready.

I've finally come to realise that how I look and dress is part of a lifetime's ambition to (unrealistically) make everything in my world appear and feel perfect. We all, to some extent, want to be seen through a flattering filter. Everyone likes a winner. Not many are happy to accept the prize for effort. (I'm sad to say this is a prize I did actually win, on the last day at my prep school, aged 11. I still have it: a copy of *Tarka The Otter*, a novel by Henry Williamson. Inside, the inscription reads: "Rose Hill School. Tunbridge Wells. Headmaster's Prize Presented To J. Langmead. For: Effort. 1977.") But what we have to accept is that perfection is beyond our reach; beyond everyone's reach. The intention behind this book is to provide you with the ability to make informed decisions about what will and what won't, or can't, make you feel better about the way you look. It's about how to look your best self, not how to look like your younger self, or even someone else.

When I was a kid I used to read a comic called *2000 AD*, home to Judge Dredd. One of the storylines revolved around a future where, due to cosmetic surgery, all the women were identical slim, button-nosed blondes (the comic reader's cliched female fantasy, basically). The twist in the tale was that everyone began to find looking "perfect" boring and unattractive and so turned to plastic surgeons to cut scars on their faces to give them a point of difference; a point of difference became more attractive than looking just like everyone else. While I don't normally turn to cartoon characters for philosophical insights, the strip made a valid point that has even more pertinence today than it did when I read it back in 1979.

Whether you love or hate this book, I hope that it proves useful. You can dismiss the entire book as utter nonsense, be thankful you're not as vain as me and potter off relieved and re-energised. Or still thank God you're not me, but find that some of the experiences resonate and some of the tips are helpful. If you want to let me know which, you can find me on Instagram @jeremylangmead. If it takes a while for me to reply it will be because I'm checking myself out in the mirror.

Part Two

By Dr David Jack

Introduction

IF YOU'D ASKED ME 18 YEARS ago when I started medical school what my eventual career would end up looking like, I certainly wouldn't have guessed I'd be doing what I am now. Initially destined for a life spent pursuing brutal reconstructive surgery in the NHS, my career has become more like that of a high-end beauty therapist – I now solely specialise in "aesthetic medicine".

Previously thought of as a hobby for doctors to make a bit of extra cash on the side to subsidise their relatively meagre NHS salaries, aesthetic medicine is fast coming of age, as the UK's governing body (the British College of Aesthetic Medicine) gradually chips away to make it a speciality in itself. Although it feels like the time since I was at medical school has passed in a flash, when we look at our attitudes towards health, ageing and beauty, there has been a marked change in the way we approach aesthetics, and the acceptability of *doing stuff* to ourselves in the name of vanity.

During the recent lockdown, I decided to watch the HBO series *The Sopranos*, having never had the time to do so before. What I found particularly entertaining was seeing how attitudes of men like Tony Soprano towards masculinity have changed significantly in the last 20 years. There are many men from backgrounds and mindsets similar to Tony among my patient cohort, but their views and the amount they are willing to spend on self-image and grooming have changed beyond recognition. I could never have imagined a Tony-Soprano type booking in for some filler back in the early 2000s (when the show was being filmed), but these days, rarely a day goes past that I don't have a few patients who fit a similar demographic.

I remember my own father's shock when he learned that one of his friends was interested in skincare and actually used some of his wife's Creme de la Mer himself in the morning. To watch his eldest son dedicate his career to skincare and wellness was doubtless not something he ever expected. But I'm pleased to say that my dad, now in his mid 60s, has a fully comprehensive skincare regime and I've even talked him into trying a bit of Botox for his crow's feet and a laser treatment for sun damage – which he actually liked, and he didn't stop telling his friends about how good he looked afterwards.

So here goes – a comprehensive rundown of the various minor cosmetic ops and treatments available, with the answers to all the questions you've ever wanted to ask. Think of it as your own private appointment with a friendly cosmetic surgeon, without the whopping bill; or perhaps more as a friendly conversation with someone in the know, who you've ended up sitting next to at a dinner party.

Tips and Treatments

IT MIGHT HELP YOU FEEL A little more in control of your dermatological destiny if you know what actually happens to you as you age. Here are some facts about the changes that occur in your face and body in each decade, from your twenties to your sixties. Apologies to anyone over 70: we've assumed you still look as if you're in your sixties, or can't see, or don't care.

What happens in each decade (and what you can choose to do about it)

Your twenties

This is when your skin is at the top of its game. The face is as full as it will ever be naturally, and lines and wrinkles are generally minimal. This is the time to look after your skin and protect it from the damage that may well be occuring already, and all the damage to come – from ultraviolet (UV) in sunlight (hopefully never sunbeds, which are an extreme and close source of damaging UV light), smoking, excessive alcohol and poor diet. All of these can have longer-term effects on the skin, so optimising your skincare and diet and having light treatments such as regular facials and maybe some gentle chemical peels (see page 196) is usually all you need to consider doing.

A major issue for some men in their twenties is adult acne, caused by a combination of hormonal changes, genetic pre-disposition, diet, stress and perhaps even imbalances of gut bacteria; it can vary from the occasional spot to a florid, severe condition. It's important to treat this early to prevent skin scar-ring over the longer term: this can be achieved with good skin-care, facials and sometimes laser treatments (see page 185).

Most people in their twenties don't need any injectable treatments. Skin boosters such as Profhilo (see pages 82 and 190) can give your skin a nice glow and are pretty low risk (and will never make you look overdone) but most men should wait until at least their thirties before going down this route.

Your thirties

This is when your face starts to lose some volume and the effects of gravity on the skin and muscles begin to show, if only marginally. How dramatic these changes are depends on a number of factors, including your genetics, ethnicity and your lifestyle so far.

At this stage in life (particularly as you approach your mid- to late-thirties), the lines and wrinkles on your face will become a little deeper and certain characteristic features, such as undereye circles, will become more pronounced. Usually a little filler and a sprinkling of Botox can help; perhaps some laser, too. I can't emphasise enough how minimal this should be in your thirties though. Looking after your skin on a daily basis with a simple but effective skincare routine should be sufficient at this stage. You do not need to invest in thousands of products, but at the very least you should use an antioxidant serum (see page 209) and an SPF (see page 210) on a daily basis to protect your skin.

Diet and healthy living is really important too, as in this decade you will find you are gradually becoming less able to still look and feel good if you burn the candle at both ends and don't look after yourself.

Your forties

There seems to be a big change as you transition from your thirties to your forties. The effects of ageing become increasingly evident on the face, as the skin begins to sag as a result of collagen damage, volume loss and the ever present pull of gravity. Drops in testosterone levels reduce the oiliness of the skin, and this combined with the effects of cumulative sun damage cause it to become thinner and less supple. Hormonal changes also contribute to hair loss from the scalp and the progressive appearance of hair in somewhat less desirable areas, particularly the ears and nostrils.

With gravity and decreasing facial volume, the overall anatomy of the face starts to change. An imbalance between the downward pulling (depressor) muscles and the upward pulling (elevator) muscles of the forehead (the frontalis) contributes to the general descent of the face. As a result, characteristic lines appear, including crow's feet at the side of the eyes, and increasingly deep frown lines. By your forties, if you're not happy with these changes, which I should say many people find perfectly attractive, you could treat them with some Botox and filler (see pages 175 and 180).

Skin thinning in the forties can be addressed quite effectively. There are some excellent biostimulating skin treatments which boost collagen and elastin levels and thicken the skin. These include skin resurfacing techniques such as CO_2 laser and fractional radiofrequency (see page 185), which create micro injuries on the skin and force the skin cells (fibroblasts) to repair the damage by increasing production of collagen and elastin, and biostimulation injectables such as Profhilo or Sculptra, (see page 189), which use chemicals to stimulate these cells.

Pre-existing sun damage to the skin is often quite apparent by your forties, with patches of hyperpigmentation and thread veins starting to appear on sun-exposed areas. These can be easily treated with laser and/or chemical peels (see pages 185 and 196) to even out skin tone and stop thread veins from becoming any bigger.

Your fifties

This decade is generally marked by fairly significant volume change in the face, a continuation of what started in earlier years. Botox and fillers can still work well (see above) but care must be taken to not over-inflate or over-freeze the face with too much of either injectable. The key to this is finding a well-trained practitioner with a good eye, who knows your face and is conservative in their approach. The face should be treated as a whole and not as individual parts (such as the cheeks, chin or jawline) which could skew or highlight particular features over others.

Volume change in the temples and forehead will become more obvious by this stage and it's likely that your eyelids will be becoming quite heavy and lax. Sometimes non-surgical options such as the plasma pen ('Plexr') may help this a little but surgery (blepharoplasty) might be a good option to reduce the skin in this area once and for all.

The sun-related damage that you noticed in your forties will also be slightly worse in your fifties, so if you've not addressed it already, laser or IPL (see page 185) is usually a simple way to do so.

Your sixties +

In your sixties your face will continue to lose volume, from the bone as well as fat and muscle. This is due to significant drops in hormone levels, reductions in your metabolic rate and changes in gene expression as a result of general DNA damage. Indeed, each time our cells divide there is a risk of DNA damage and of changes to our genes; the older we get, the more likely we are to see some abnormal gene expression and "senescence" (ageing of our cells). The way these changes manifest in our skin is as thinning and collagen loss. All features of facial ageing are obvious by the time we hit our sixties and the question at this stage tends to be: "Should

I be having a little nip and tuck?" Often the effectiveness of filler and Botox for lifting is limited by now, so surgery is the only option if you're really not happy.

But do men do facelifts? And doesn't it feminise the face? The answer is yes to the former (in recent years it has become a lot more common) and no to the latter – provided it's done properly by someone who has experience in treating male faces. The technique for a masculine facelift is different from that for a woman, unless it's for gender reassignment. With men's facelifts, it's very important to maintain as much facial width, with no slimming or thinning of the jawline; for this reason, extent of lifting is usually less in men than it is in women. Similarly, the position and pattern of the surgical incision is of particular importance as most men tend to have shorter hair (or perhaps no hair at all), making the scar more difficult to hide. As sideburns need to be maintained in their normal position in men, the usual "pre-auricular" incisions (i.e. in front of the ear) have to be carefully edited so that the scars are camouflaged within them. Most people don't want either hairy earlobes or no sideburns. Men's skin is generally heavier than women's, too, so the expectations for the eventual healed outcome are usually more conservative.

If you're not into the idea of surgery, then some gentle revolumisation with filler and wrinkle relaxation with Botox is certainly still an option. Lasers and skin resurfacing can also remain fairly effective in later life. I've got some patients in their nineties who still come to me for Botox and fillers and find it makes a difference when they compare themselves to their facially unedited peers.

Here's the skinny on eight unscary, non-invasive treatments that both Jeremy and I have tried and hand-on-heart recommend.

——————— 1 ———————
WHAT YOU CAN DO FOR FINE LINES AND WRINKLES

Botox

What does it do?

Without doubt, the best-known non-surgical treatment on the market is Botox cosmetic. It was launched over 30 years ago, and yet I still see first-time patients who come in convinced that they will look like they have been through a wind tunnel if they have this treatment. I'd like to assure you that the reality nowadays is very different. The key to success is to use it to relax (not freeze) facial lines and to inject enough but not too much so that the muscle maintains a bit of movement.

When I first started doing Botox around 13 years ago (both for patients and also on myself!), I'd say around 10% of my patients were men. Nowadays, the number of male patients has more than doubled, and includes men from all walks of life and income levels. "Having their Botox done" is now almost like having a trim at the barber's every few months for many men, and the stigma attached to it is really starting to subside.

What's in it?

The description of Botox is a bit of a misnomer as the doses that are injected for cosmetic treatments are not anywhere near a level that would be described as "toxic" – the "toxic" effects on the body only come from infection with the bacterium *Clostridium botulinum*, in which large amounts of the protein it produces can wreak havoc on the muscular system. In cosmetic treatments, microdoses of this protein can be injected directly into muscles, causing them to temporarily relax. The protein does this by blocking the nerve signals from the brain telling the muscle fibres to contract. This muscle relaxation in turn relaxes the lines on the skin that the muscles of facial expression have created over the years. There is usually a time lag of 3–5 days between having injections and the effects beginning to show and then about two weeks before they are fully visible.

There are a number of brands of botulinum toxin on the market, the best known of which is the one manufactured by Allergan, called Botox. Other brands include Dysport, Xeomin and Bocouture. Dosing is slightly different for each, and each practitioner will have their preference. My favourite is the original Allergan Botox as it has the longest and most extensive clinical data and is very predictable in its mechanism of action.

Why it's okay

A big part of skin ageing relates to the effects of gravity and gradual imbalances in the relative strength of the different facial muscles. Over time, the downward pulling depressor muscles become stronger than the lifting elevator muscles (as they have fewer forces to overcome). This, in combination with changes in the skin quality over the years, and volume change in the face, can cause the face to sag in certain very predicatable areas, and the skin to form deep grooves as it loses collagen and elastin. In the past, when Botox was first available, doctors tended to go wild with dosing, completely paralysing both the depressor and elevator muscles. This had the effect of disrupting the normal muscular architecture of the face and resulted in some very odd appearances. Nowadays, minimal, strategic dosing can relax the problematic lines without doing this.

When to use it

Botox for the *prevention* of line formation is somewhat overkill in my opinion. The best time to start having it is when you're starting to see some fine lines when your face is at rest. In most people, this will be in the mid-thirties, as collagen levels start to drop and the skin has slightly less resilience to the forces of the muscles pulling on it. If you start with a small dose of Botox at this stage the lines won't progress as much as they would normally and you may need less over time for maintenance.

The areas of the face that are most commonly treated with Botox are the frown lines (or "glabella"), the forehead lines and the crow's feet ("lateral canthal lines"). However, with experienced practitioners, it can be used to reverse muscular imbalances and lines elsewhere on the face and neck, such as a depressed nasal tip, mouth to chin "marionette" lines and sagging of the jaw and neck – the latter treatment is sometimes called the "Nefertiti lift". For this, Botox is injected under the chin and down the neck in about 20–25 points across the platysma muscle (the muscle that forms the strong neck bands you will see if you grimace). It's a relatively quick and painless procedure that can produce a very subtle lifting effect on the jawline, reducing the vertical bands you often see developing with age, and also helps (in some cases) to lift the fat pad under the chin.

Jawline bulkiness caused by the big chewing muscles on the sides of the face can be treated with Botox, too. In fact, injections into the masseter muscles on the sides of the face can, over time, slim this muscle. In addition, they have been shown to reduce teeth grinding.

Botox also works on the nerves that cause sweating, which has led to its use in treating a condition known as hyperhidrosis, where excess perspiration can be quite problematic.

What to avoid

The major thing to avoid with Botox is overdosing. With a good, experienced practitioner, your Botox should always just make it look as if you've had a good sleep and are well rested, with open eyes and supple skin. You should also be able to make dynamic movements (i.e. still make facial expressions). If you can't move your muscles at all after Botox, it's a sign that you have probably had too much (or that you are particularly sensitive to it). Fret not – it will wear off, but it is likely to take a few months. The best approach is to have a small dose that can be topped up after the two-week period it takes to be fully effective, rather than accept a whacking dose and risk having your muscles rendered totally (if temporarily) paralysed. If your friends specifically ask if you've had Botox, it might be a sign to put the brakes on.

Inexperienced, untrained practitioners don't have the detailed appreciation of facial anatomy that comes from training at medical school. I would always say to go for an experienced doctor, surgeon, nurse prescriber or dentist (yes – dentists are often good Botox practitioners as they have generally done a lot of facial-anatomy training). You should never ever let a beauty therapist inject your face with Botox. It is a prescription medication with potential side effects. Unfortunately, in the UK, current legislation allows any practitioner to perform the treatment (provided Botox has been prescribed by a doctor) but is majorly risky. At the end of the day, this is your face! It's worth spending a little more to have things done properly. And don't be tempted by cut-price offers – I'd be concerned about the skill of a practitioner who has to market to people based on price.

How long is the recovery?

Although there is a tiny risk of bruising with any injectable treatment, and Botox may cause a mild headache on the day it is done, the recovery is short and straightforward. For 5–10 minutes after a treatment, you may have some small bumps under the skin at the injection points, due to the fluid that the Botox is diluted in. Don't worry, it dissipates very quickly. Tiny dots of blood might also appear on the injection sites but these can be wiped off with some antiseptic. For the first hour after the treatment, I'd recommend that you don't lie flat; some practitioners say that you shouldn't exercise for 24 hours, but there isn't any clinical evidence for this.

How long does it last?

The lifespan of the treatment varies from person to person, depending on the dose and other factors, such as the starting strength of their muscles. Botox should last 3–4 months, but in some people who are very active it may last as little as two months, while in others I've seen it lasting almost a year!

2
WHAT YOU CAN DO FOR VOLUME LOSS

Dermal fillers

The idea of fillers for men who are fresh to the world of aesthetics can sometimes be a little scary. The concern is that you risk ending up looking like a feminised alien, and that there is no going back once you have started. Thankfully, the reality is that this is very rarely the case – the fillers we use nowadays are generally reversible if you don't like them. And all properly trained doctors will know enough about proportions to avoid making you look as if you've just landed from a distant galaxy.

What do they do?

Over time, we all lose facial volume. The bony skeleton of the face (like every other bone in the body) is in a state of constant renewal. To explain this in a little more detail: throughout our lives, our bones undergo a process known as bone turnover, in which they are constantly broken down and then remade in order to maintain our calcium levels (since bone is essentially a reservoir of calcium). As we age, the rate at which new bone is produced drops below the rate at which it is made, so the overall volume of bone decreases. This happens mostly on the surfaces of facial bones, so in effect they progressively move inwards, causing the eye sockets to widen, the cheekbones to lose projection and the jawline to become slimmer. This is a very gradual process – it's pretty much impossible to notice over the short term, but over the longer term the loss of bony volume in the face causes the overlying fat and skin to start to lose support and sag downwards, with the pull of gravity. Alongside bony-volume loss, facial fat also loses volume over time and the other support tissues become increasingly lax. This results in the formation of deep grooves, thinning lips, jowls and general drooping of the face.

What fillers do best is replace volume where it's been lost. The key to good fillers is finding a skilled practitioner who really knows and appreciates the anatomical changes that happen over time to the face, and can add tiny amounts of filler to the areas that predictably lose volume the most.

What are they?

Fillers have been around for decades. They are injectable substances which add volume to tissues without creating an immune reaction. A number of different substances can be used as fillers but by far the most common is the molecule known as hyaluronic acid. Hyaluronic acid basically comprises long chains of proteins and sugars that attract water molecules to themselves. This is what can cause the small risk of swelling after the procedure and, if too much filler has been used, a puffy appearance to the face.

Fillers are injected under the skin, either onto the surface of the bone, or into the fatty tissue of the face (or even elsewhere in the body, such as the bottom or hands) with a tiny needle or a "cannula" (a longer blunt needle with an opening on the side of the tip). The choice of technique will depend on your practitioner's preference and experience.

The nice thing about hyaluronic acid is that it can be broken down by the enzyme hyaluronidase (hyalase), so if you don't like the effect, it can be remedied.

Which brands to use

The best filler brands should all be FDA-approved in the US and CE-marked in the EU. They are classified as "medical devices", so don't necessarily need a prescription, but I'd always advise seeing a doctor, dentist or even an experienced nurse prescriber for any filler procedure. Most good brands come with local anaesthetic mixed into the filler so the treatment is a fairly painless one.

Why they're okay

Generally speaking, filler is pretty much suitable for anyone, unless you have a rare sensitivity to certain cross linking agents used in them, which is very unusual.

In which areas of the face can you have fillers?

To create an overall harmonious lifting effect that looks normal, your doctor should look at your face as a whole – not just particular areas such as the cheeks or jawline. A big issue with some less-experienced or non-medical practitioners is that they tend to offer stand-alone treatments such as cheek fillers or lip fillers – almost trying to play God by creating structures that wouldn't naturally be found on your face, in turn disrupting the normal facial proportions. Fillers should be used to replace lost volume in multiple areas of the face in a minimalistic, more general way – "always replace, don't create" is the mantra.

That said, a number of areas are particularly suited to

revolumisation with filler, including the jawline, undereye (or "tear trough") area, mid face, temples and even the nose. Indeed, "non-surgical rhinoplasty" (the nose job) has become increasingly popular over the last few years.

When to stop

Any good doctor will stop you from going too far, so it's important to choose your practitioner wisely – personal recommendations from friends (those who look good!) are always the best.

How long is the recovery and what are the risks?

Recovery from fillers is pretty minimal. Even straight after the treatment, there are often no signs you've had anything done, provided the correct volumes are injected. There is a tiny risk of bruising (as with any injection into the face) which can last for a few days, swelling for 24–48 hours (this can be more on one side of the face than the other) and a tiny risk of skin damage secondary to injection into a blood vessel and blockage (known as a "vascular occlusion"). This is extremely rare but needs to be treated immediately with the enzyme hyaluronidase to remove the filler and restore the blood flow to the skin. Any medical practitioner should be able to recognise the signs of vascular occlusion and treat it – this is a major reason for not going to a non-medically trained injector.

How long do they last?

Hyaluronic acid is constantly turned over in the skin, so over a period of 6–18 months (depending on the brand and type of filler used), the filler will be broken down by the body and usually completely disappear. If you continue to have the procedure done over a longer period of time, you generally find that you need to add less volume each time as there is some left over. The ideal is that eventually you grow some permanent collagen and elastin tissue that replaces the filler and creates more permanent volume.

3

WHAT TO DO WHEN YOU START TO NOTICE YOUR SKIN AGEING

Lasers, energy-based treatments, skin resurfacing and skin tightening

What are they?

As the skin ages, the dermis (the thick supportive layer of the skin) gets thinner and progressively more lax as it loses collagen, elastin and other structural molecules. There is a constant turnover throughout life of these molecules, with resynthesis by the skin's fibroblasts increasingly being lost in favour of breakdown. Genetic factors, UV damage and lifestyle influences such as smoking, stress and poor diet are all to blame. Sun damage results not only in thinning but also in pigmentation changes and increased redness as the thin skin allows the superficial blood vessels to show through.

Over the last 20 or so years, a number of biostimulating treatments have been developed to address the changes that occur in the different layers of the skin. These include skin boosters (such as Profhilo, which will be covered in the next section) and energy-based treatments, which include lasers, fractional resurfacing (intense pulsed light), and high intensity focused ultrasound (HIFU).

How do they work?

Lasers, IPL and other energy-based treatments including fractional resurfacing and HIFU, use different types of energy to create certain effects, cleverly utilising the skin's natural physiology to reverse some of the changes that happen over the years.

Lasers and IPL use very strong sources of light energy, either of a single wavelength (laser) or blended wavelengths of light (IPL), to target specific coloured molecules in the skin (known as chromophores) or water. Once these molecules absorb the light, it causes them to vibrate, heat up and either be destroyed or vapourised. In this way, lasers and IPL can be used to target issues such as brown pigmentation and red thread veins.

CO_2 laser is an example of fractional resurfacing (meaning a treatment that creates micro injuries to a fraction of the skin surface). Radiofrequency microneedling (such as Fractora, Morpheus8 or INTRAcel), and standard microneedling techniques (such as derma roller or dermapen) all also work on this principle. Both radiofrequency (RF) microneedling and standard microneedling use physical pins to create these microinjuries – the latter boosting the physical microinjuries by delivering radiofrequency energy through the needles. This in turn stimulates a healing response in the skin, thickening the dermis layer and increasing the production of new collagen and elastin during the months post-treatment. Radiofrequency microneedling has a more potent effect compared to standard microneedling without radiofrequency.

HIFU devices such as Ultherapy or Ultracel use a different type of energy to fractionally injure tiny areas of the muscle layer below the skin, and, over time, bring about a lifting and tightening of the deep tissues of the face as it heals.

Why they're okay

For people averse to the idea of injecting substances into the skin, lasers and energy-based treatments offer the opportunity to reverse some of the signs of ageing in a more "natural" way. There is practically no risk of looking odd with laser treatments, unless you are unfortunate enough to get a burn (which is rare). Treatments that heat the deeper tissues of the face, such as HIFU, may cause some reduction in the fat volume, but this isn't common.

When to use them

I'd always suggest speaking to a well-experienced laser practitioner before you consider any energy-based skin treatment. There are so many devices on the market and every clinic will try to persuade you that their device is the best. Clinics with many lasers and experienced practitioners, should be able to advise on what will work best for your particular issue and make a suitable treatment plan.

Most laser and energy treatments will require a course rather than a single treatment.

How long is the recovery?

Recovery from lasers, energy-based treatments and fractional resurfacing varies according to the particular device and also the energy settings that are used. Risks are low but there is a slight risk of burns with any energy-based treatment. For laser, a test patch should be offered before treatment to check your skin isn't going to react. For people with darker skin types, lasers and IPL should be administered with caution, and by experienced hands. A rough guide to recovery times would be as follows:

IPL: 1–2 days of mild redness and sensitivity, 7 days of darkening of pigment and potentially bruising if thread veins were present (these lighten after this time as the pigment and clotted blood is removed by the body).

Fractional lasers, e.g. Fraxel: around 4–7 days of redness, mild swelling and sometimes scabbing.

Fractional radiofrequency e.g. Morpheus8: around 1–2

days of mild redness, roughness of the skin for up to a week and mild swelling for the first day or so.

Microneedling, e.g. derma roller: redness and mild swelling for a day or so.

How long do they last?

This really depends on the type of treatment. The effects of IPL for hyperpigmentation, for example, usually last for a year or two, whereas fractional radiofrequency or HIFU only need to be repeated every five years or so.

Are there any less-invasive alternatives?

Other energy-based treatments, such as non-ablative radiofrequency (for example Thermage, Forma or Pellevé), heat the skin more gently, without creating micro injuries. These treatments are good for gentle lifting but usually require many sessions to make a real difference.

—————— *4* ——————

SKIN BOOSTERS

What are they?

The new kids on the block in the world of aesthetic treatments are skin boosters. These are injectable treatments that are designed to brighten and improve the quality of the skin in a gentler, more "natural" way. The concept behind them is the principle of mesotherapy, developed by Dr Michel Pistor in France in the 1950s. Mesotherapy continues to be a popular treatment to this day as a way of imbuing the skin with a freshness and gently reducing fine lines and wrinkles; but in recent years more advanced skin boosters such as Profhilo, Juvedérm Volite and Teosyal Redensity 1 have stolen the show.

Another type of treatment, known as platelet-rich plasma (PRP) involves injecting plasma isolated from a sample of your own blood into your skin, and is thought to have a biostimulating effect.

What do they do?

Most skin booster treatments contain a blend of molecules in a fluid form that is injected fairly superficially into the skin. Mesotherapy often contains a mix of vitamins, micronutrients and hyaluronic acid, whereas treatments such as Profhilo and Juvéderm Volite contain only hyaluronic acid, and in high quantities. Despite being made of the same basic molecules, Profhilo, Volite and other skin boosters are generally not considered to be "fillers" as such; and indeed, they act in a quite different way. Profhilo, in particular, does not contain the dense chemical links ("crosslinks") between the molecules which turn them into a gel, meaning it doesn't actually add any volume to the tissues, but acts instead as a hydrator and also as a biostimulator – forcing the skin to ramp up its production of new collagen and elastin over a 3–6 month period following the treatment, by virtue of the free-floating hyaluronic acid molecules. Teosyal Redensity 1 is similar to this, whereas Juvéderm Volite is slightly more crosslinked, so has some of the characteristics of a filler but the volume added will always be fairly minimal.

Mesotherapy injections can brighten and hydrate dull skin and with prolonged and repeated use they are believed, like Profhilo, to stimulate the cells of the dermis to produce new collagen and elastin.

With PRP, a sample of your blood is taken and put in a centrifuge machine to separate the different components of the blood into layers. The plasma and platelet parts of the blood are then isolated and siphoned off into a syringe for reinjection into the skin. Reinjecting them into the skin triggers a process known as "platelet degranulation", in which the the growth factors contained within the platelets are released (this is what happens naturally in the body when platelets are activated in areas of inflammation). These growth factors, when released in high quantities, are thought to stimulate the fibroblasts in the skin to increase their activity and produce more collagen and elastin fibres. This in turn can reduce fine lines and wrinkles over a period of several months.

Why they're okay

Skin boosters, unlike Botox or filler, are quite difficult to do badly. The risk of side effects, and looking weird if they are overdone, is very low. Pretty much everyone's skin will benefit from skin boosters – they are a nice way to gently improve the quality of the skin as we age.

What is the treatment like?

Mesotherapy is a particularly gentle treatment; although it uses needles, the injections are often so superficial that they don't cause any pain or bleeding. Profhilo and other skin boosters involve slightly deeper injections, which can sting a little.

PRP is often done in combination with microneedling, which creates redness and sometimes swelling for a few hours, but it is not particularly painful.

When to use

Skin boosters can be administered fairly frequently. Mesotherapy is generally done once per month, whereas skin boosters like Profhilo usually involve a pattern of two initial treatments, one month apart, then either once every three months or two sessions every 6–9 months. Juvéderm Volite and other skin boosters are similar.

How long do they last?

The effects from these treatments vary and with regular sessions there will be some degree of longer-term benefit to the skin. For example, mesotherapy is quick to take effect and usually brightens and hydrates the skin for about a month, but it requires regular repeating to show much benefit in the long term.

PRP and Profhilo, which are thought to be much more potent collagen and elastin stimulators, work over a much longer term, so the results are slower to show (they usually take six months or more), but last for longer.

——————————— 5 ———————————

NON-SURGICAL FAT REDUCTION

What are the options?

Although the obvious thing to do if you're feeling a little podgy might be to amend your diet and start on a training programme, for some men, a quicker and easier fix is more appealing. Over the last few years, a number of techniques have evolved, both in terms of non-surgical treatments and minimally invasive surgery. These usually work best for stubborn pockets of fat rather than massive weight loss, and are often used after you've got some weight off through a programme of diet and exercise and just want to help shift the last little bit.

Surgery (liposuction and skin reduction techniques such as abdominoplasty or tummy-tuck) was the go-to in the 1990s, but these days most people will try less-invasive options before going down that route.

How does it work?

Most non-surgical fat reduction techniques work on the basis that fat cells are pretty unstable and sensitive to changes in temperature and certain chemicals. A number of treatments have evolved using these principles, of which probably the best known is cryolipolysis or fat freezing. This involves attaching a chilling machine onto an area of fat with suction, which freezes the tissue for 35–70 minutes at around -9 Celsius, stimulating permanent death of about 30% of the fat cells (but not the skin, muscle or nerve cells) in a given area. Usually you'd repeat the treatment twice or three times for the best results.

A couple of alternatives to fat freezing are also gaining popularity. These include fat-busting injections, made from a chemical called deoxycholic acid (brands include Aqualyx, Celluform and Kybella), which is selectively toxic to fat cells (meaning that it doesn't do much to any other cell type). Another treatment involves the injection of heated carbon dioxide gas, which is similarly selectively toxic to these cells. The latter is known as carboxytherapy. Usually you'd have two to three deoxycholic acid injections in a given area, about a month apart. Carboxytherapy is a weekly treatment that requires 10–12 sessions, so is a bit more time-consuming.

What are the risks?

All of these treatments are pretty safe and relatively effective; however, they have a knock-on effect on the skin, which risks becoming slightly loose as the fat beneath it is reduced. This can be remedied with skin-tightening treatments such as fractional resurfacing or radiofrequency heating, which I have described earlier in the section on lasers and energy-based treatments (see page 185). The body usually requires longer treatments than the face as the tissues targeted are deeper beneath the surface.

In a tiny percentage of patients (under 0.0051%), fat freezing has been shown to result in the opposite of the desired outcome, i.e. the fat cells actually gain volume, in a syndrome known as paradoxical adipose hyperplasia. This has to be treated with liposuction. It is very rare, and just something to be aware of.

Deoxycholic acid is very safe to use but there is a small risk of lumpiness after treatments, which usually resolves over time. Bruising and swelling happen in almost all cases. This is especially important to note if you're planning to have it for treatment of a double chin – deoxycholic acid gives a bit of a frog-like appearance for about two weeks.

As for carboxytherapy, there is a risk of bruising and very temporary swelling (often no more than an hour).

N.B. Gynaecomastia

Although we are not recommending any surgical procedures here, I'm often asked by clients about treatment for gynaecomastia (i.e. the development of male breast tissue). It's a very common issue, and can be psychologically challenging for men who are affected, often causing them to opt for cosmetic surgery. Hormone changes, use of anabolic steroids, genes and high body fat are all factors that may contribute to the development of this condition. In most cases of gynaecomastia, there will be very minimal actual glandular breast tissue and largely just fat cells.

A number of different techniques are available for treating gynaecomastia, the choice of which depends on the surgeon and the amount of tissue involved. Often liposuction is used in combination with excision (i.e. cutting out) of glandular tissue if there is any present. The procedure sometimes involves an incision around the areola of the nipple. Nipple inversion (where the nipple has the appearance of being pulled in) can also be corrected.

The procedure is done under a local or general anaesthetic, depending on the indiviudal case. Recovery is fairly quick, with just some swelling and bruising, for which a compression garment is often worn for a week or so. If a cut is made around the areola, stitches are usually removed after 10–14 days. The risks involved in the reduction of gynaecomastia are similar to those with liposuction, infection and seroma formation very occasionally being an issue.

6

SKIN PEELS

I get some terrified looks in clinic when I suggest that a patient has a skin peel. The automatic assumption is that your skin will be falling off in chunks and you will be left with red skin for weeks afterwards. In reality, this is very far from the truth.

As it happens, most chemical peels for home use are fairly gentle and offer a great way to refresh your skin every so often. Peeling usually refers to products that exfoliate the skin, i.e. they strip back some of the surface layers. At-home products have lower concentrations of active ingredients than in-clinic peels but can include similar acids such as alpha-hydroxy acids (AHAs, such as glycolic, mandelic or lactic acid), azelaic acid, retinoids (Vitamin A) and vitamin C. Generally speaking, these can be used more regularly than clinic-based treatments and will cause very little downtime or side effects. In-clinic treatments can also feature stronger ingredients such as tricholoracetic acid (TCA) and phenol that need to be handled by professionals as the risk of side effects such as burns and irritation is higher.

What are the benefits of peeling and exfoliation?

Not only does exfoliation make your skin look brighter (since it removes some of its dead layers), but it can also help regular daily skincare products penetrate deeper and more effectively. Peels can also contain ingredients that have a specific purpose – for example ingredients to treat hyperpigmentation or scarring, or to limit active acne.

Another way of exfoliating, without using any chemicals, is to physically exfoliate. Physical exfoliation products contain granules of hard, inert substances that can basically rub away the top layers of the skin (the epidermis). Some people like these sort of products – not me. Physical exfoliation is a bit rough on the skin surface and might even cause more inflammation, so I usually recommend my patients use chemical exfoliants.

Another increasingly popular in-clinic exfoliating treatment is dermaplaning, which involves physically exfoliating the skin with a surgical blade. This treatment has exploded in the last few years on social media with the introduction of many home kits. While this technique might seem easy and straightforward enough to do at home, it has to be performed in a particular way for best results and is therefore usually best left to a trained professional.

How often can I exfoliate the skin?

My recommendation for gentle chemical exfoliation at home is once a week. Just be aware that, if your skin is sensitive, over-exfoliation can exacerbate this and cause redness and dryness. For in-clinic superficial-depth peels, I'd usually say once every six weeks (i.e. once every skin cycle) is more than enough to balance risks vs benefits, and for deeper peels much less frequently. Dermaplaning can be done in-clinic every 4–6 weeks.

How long should I leave a peel on my skin?

Although home peels are meant to be designed so they can be left on the skin safely for longer than indicated without risking major damage, I'd always recommend sticking to the instructions for your individual products to avoid any doubt. In-clinic-strength peels available online are not a good idea. Just don't buy them.

Do I need to wash peels off?

Not always. Some products are designed to be left on and will self-neutralise, while others need to be washed off. Stronger products (particularly higher-strength glycolic acids) might need to be treated with a neutraliser. Always follow the instructions on your individual product.

Aren't chemical peels risky?

This really depends on the depth of peel and your own skin. The stronger and deeper a peel is, the higher the risk of any side effects. Peels need to be treated with respect and not overdone but, if you use them as directed, side effects are rare. If you get some redness or heightened sensitivity, you should speak to a skincare specialist or dermatologist.

One drawback of certain peeling ingredients is that they can heighten your sun sensitivity. This is usually due to the ingredients themselves as well as the fact that they reduce the protective barrier of the skin. It's essential to wear a broad-spectrum high-factor SPF after any sort of exfoliation.

Which chemicals are in chemical peels?

In terms of individual peeling ingredients that can be used in home products, the list is extensive. The following are the most frequently used ingredients, and they are generally available at stronger concentrations in in-clinic peels.

Alpha-hydroxy acids (AHAs)

These are a group of water-soluble organic acids. The most commonly found forms in skincare are:

- *Glycolic acid* – derived from sugar cane, glycolic acid is one of the most popular AHAs in home products. It is suitable for use at up to about 10% in home products – higher-strength versions may need to be washed off or neutralised. It is a fantastic exfoliant, which helps unclog pores and can also reduce hyperpigmentation and acne

- *Lactic acid* – slightly weaker than glycolic acid, lactic acid (as its name suggests) is derived from milk. It has been used in various forms for centuries as an exfoliant and pigment corrector. It can also reduce acne and inflammation, and has been shown to help the skin stay hydrated by stimulating ceramide formation (the natural fatty acids that help the skin retain moisture).

- *Mandelic acid* – a slightly gentler AHA than others in the group, mandelic acid is derived from bitter almonds. It is good for exfoliation and on acne, but has the strongest effects on hyperpigmentation. In one study, regular use of mandelic acid for four weeks reduced pigmentation by 50% vs the control group. It is a large molecule, so doesn't penetrate the skin quite as deeply as others.

- *Citric acid* – you've guessed it, this AHA is derived from citrus fruits, such as lemons, oranges and limes. Citric acid is commonly used in skincare as a pH balancer and preservative. It is an exfoliant and can brighten the skin, although its effects tend to be less powerful than those of other AHAs.

- *Tartaric acid* – this AHA is derived from fermented grapes. It is often used in combination with other AHAs to help balance their pHs and increase their effectiveness.

- *Malic acid* – derived primarily from apples, this AHA is slightly weaker than others but still has some exfoliating and brightening effects. It is often used in combination with another AHA for best results.

- *Phytic acid* – a weak AHA, phytic acid is mostly used to reduce waxy sebum in the skin, caused by high calcium levels, which make the natural oils become thicker. Phytic acid works to chelate (i.e. soak up) the excess calcium and reduce this, so it can be great for unclogging pores and reducing blackheads. It is also an antioxidant and can help reduce hyperpigmentation.

Beta-hydroxy acid (BHA)

- *Salicylic acid* – slightly different in structure than the AHAs, beta-hydroxy acid or salicylic acid is a potent exfoliator, anti-inflammatory and anti-bacterial derived from willow bark (it's also used to make aspirin). As it is fat soluble, it can penetrate deep into the pores, making it a top choice for treating acne, blocked pores and blackheads. However, salicylic acid can be quite drying, and overuse can actually lead to a condition called salicylate poisoning, so don't use it over your whole body at any one time!

Poly-hydroxy acids

These are the new generation of AHAs that have been developed to be slightly less irritating on the skin. They generally have larger molecules so don't penetrate deeply but still have similar exfoliating and brightening effects. They provide photoprotection (i.e. can prevent some UV damage to the skin over time) and also act as iron chelators, meaning they can reduce the ageing, oxidative effects produced by iron. Examples of PHAs include:

- *Gluconolactone* – this PHA is a powerful antioxidant. It can prevent thinning of the skin by inhibiting the enzyme elastase, which breaks down the skin's elastin molecules over time. It also helps hydrate the skin by repairing its natural barrier and by producing its own humectant (moisturising) effect.

- *Lactobionic acid* – similar to gluconolactone, this acid derived from milk sugar is a powerful humectant. It is a gentle exfoliator and can brighten the skin, reduce hyper-pigmentation and improve texture. It can also improve skin firmness by blocking collagen and elastin breakdown

Dicarboxylic acids

These are a group of acids used in peels and a range of other skincare products for their antioxidant, anti-inflammatory and hydrating effects.

- *Azelaic acid* – the most commonly used dicarboxylic acid found in skincare, azelaic acid was traditionally derived from wheat, barley and rye. It has flown under the radar for a long time in the skincare world. Something of a powerhouse, it has potent antioxidant, antibacterial and hydrating effects on the skin. It can help fade pigmentation, repair the skin's barrier and is increasingly a top choice for treating rosacea. It is gently exfoliating so can unclog pores but is less harsh than most AHAs and BHA.

Alpha-keto acids

- *Pyruvic acid* – a relative newcomer to home peeling, pyruvic acid can help reduce sebum production, reduce hyperpigmentation and stimulate collagen production. It is generally used only in-clinic.

Hydroxycinnamic acids

These acids are found in plant cell walls and are potent antioxidants.

- *Ferulic acid* – the number one hydroxycinnamic acid in skincare, ferulic acid is often used in combination with vitamins C and E for its synergistic antioxidant effects (i.e. one boosts the activity of another). It is a top choice for pigmentation reduction and anti-ageing.

- *Retinoic acid (vitamin A)* – one of the key ingredients in modern, active skincare, higher-strength retinoids can be used in peels for both their exfoliating effects and also to reduce pigmentation and sebum production for people suffering from acne. See the next section on skincare routine for a full overview of retinoids.

- *Ascorbic acid (vitamin C)* – the chief antioxidant in many skincare formulations, vitamin C, has fantastic anti-ageing, collagen-stimulating and pigmentation-reducing effects on the skin. Higher doses can be used intermittently in peels/weekly exfoliators to give an extra powerful effect. As I've mentioned earlier in the chapter on antioxidants, when combined with vitamin E and ferulic acid, as well as other ingredients like glutathione, the effects of vitamin C can be heightened

Clinic-only ingredients

Some peeling agents are too strong or unstable to be used in home products but can have some very dramatic effects on the skin if used correctly. They tend to have a higher risk of side effects such as redness and physical peeling, so should only be used by trained practitioners. These include:

- *Trichloroacetic acid (TCA)*

- *Phenol*

Beware of any home peels containing these ingredients!

--------- 7 ---------

THE BENEFITS OF A SKINCARE ROUTINE

Like any other organ of the body, the skin needs a little maintenance on a regular basis. This is particularly so if you have a skin condition such as acne or rosacea. It's not an overnight thing. With progress in skincare technology and advances in the understanding of the benefits of active ingredients (i.e. those that have distinct effects on the skin), choosing the right products is much more straightforward now. But most active skincare products take a while to show any results, so I always encourage patients to choose a regime and stick to it for at least a few months (unless it's causing any issues).

With so many suggested skincare regimes out there, deciding what is best for you can be quite an overwhelming task. It's always a good idea when you're considering a new regime to speak to a skin specialist (whether they are an aesthetician, cosmetic doctor or dermatologist) and ideally have them design one specifically suited to you. It's important for them to take a close look at your skin, as well as a thorough history of it, and of your general health. Skincare is by no means a one-fits-all business but there are certainly some things we will all benefit from, regardless of age or gender.

For any skincare regime, I would recommend keeping things as simple as possible, firstly so you can remember the steps easily (so they become second nature), and secondly so you reduce the risk of any interactions or irritation.

A good way of starting a new regime is by looking at what you are currently using and performing an edit. Do you really need three serums, an SPF, two moisturisers and a separate mist? I'd say an absolute maximum of five good-quality, core products should be enough for anyone's skin for a daily routine.

The principles of good skincare are based on science, and take into account the layers, acidity and penetration of any skincare product and the evidence behind the ingredients being used. Before you go out and spend a huge amount of money on some newly advertised product, remember that there is a limit to what we can actually do with topical skincare. My message to you is: be sensible, always question why you're using something and be selective. Your skin is a homeostatic organ, meaning it regulates its own function most of the time.

The main categories of skincare to include in your regime, in my opinion, are as follows:

- *Cleanser* – to clean the skin and remove debris.

- *Exfoliator* – to help products penetrate the skin.

- *Antioxidant serum* – to neutralise free radicals (that cause skin or chemical damage).

- *Sunscreen* – to protect the skin against UV damage.

- *Specific ingredients* – to address any individual issue, e.g. additional moisturiser for dry skin, or something for hyperpigmentation.

- *Dietary supplement* – to boost the skin from inside (see next section).

As one product can often fit into multiple categories, you don't necessarily need six products. When your practitioner is designing your regime, they will have these principles in mind, so it is good to understand their rationale in whatever they tell you to use. In the following section, I'm going to go through some of these categories in turn to explain what they are and when and how you should use them.

Cleansers

"Cleanliness is next to godliness" goes the saying. Is this the case with skincare, though? Well, to an extent, but we don't need to overdo it. Our skin comes in contact with environmental pollutants, dirt and other chemicals on a daily basis. Particulate matter can block pores and even stimulate inflammation in the skin, so it needs to be washed off before we even think about applying other products. We need to go carefully, though: we have a particularly important group of bacteria living on our skin surface, which help keep our skin's barrier function intact and without which we become prone to irritation and a variety of skin conditions.

Many of the environmental impurities and cosmetic products are not water soluble, so washing the skin with water alone would be insufficient to remove them. To address this, cleansers contain substances that emulsify these particles, i.e. make them water soluble. An ideal cleanser should remove the day's grime and make-up, without damaging or irritating the skin; it should also try to keep the skin surface moist. It is known that overly drying cleansers can cause damage to the skin barrier, leading to disruption, irritation and inflammation.

A number of different types of cleanser are on the market, including the following:

- *Micellar waters* – these are clear fluids containing "micelles", which are essentially little fat pockets that can emulsify any fat-soluble debris on the skin (including make-up).

- *Gel and foam liquid cleansers* – this type of cleanser foams and produces a lather. Often these products contain active ingredients such as acids (e.g. AHAs/BHA) to help manage oily and acne-prone skin, providing a mild exfoliation as well as cleansing, and other antioxidants.

- *Cream and lotion cleansers* – creams (thicker consistency) and lotions (thinner) are good for removing bulky debris such as make-up from the skin. They are often formulated with emollients such as glycerin or shea butter, and are hydrating and soothing on the skin. Creams and lotions tend to be the favourite choice for people with dry skin or those who suffer from inflammation or redness.

- *Oil cleansers* – putting oils on your face might not seem like a sensible thing to do when you're trying to clean your skin but oil cleansers actually dissolve a lot of the fat-soluble debris and sebum that collects on it during the day. These are popular with people with sensitive skin conditions such as rosacea who might have a disrupted epidermal barrier.

- ***Balm and melting balm cleansers*** – these are rich butter-like formulations that melt when applied to the skin. They can usually be used without water to dissolve dirt, sweat and make-up and are generally very soothing.

Exfoliators

I've discussed skin peels in section 6 but a mention should be given to exfoliators in your home skincare routine. Exfoliating has a number of benefits in addition to those of its individual ingredients, including improving penetration of active skincare products and enhancing the skin's normal bacteria by regulating its pH. Examples of exfoliating ingredients in skincare include AHAs, such as glycolic, lactic, mandelic and phytic acid, beta-hydroxy acid (also known as salicylic acid) and azelaic acid. If you have particularly sensitive skin, I'd say opt for exfoliators that are going to be gentle, such as azelaic and mandelic acids, rather than the slightly more aggressive glycolic or beta-hydroxy acid, which may cause redness and irritation. If your skin is particularly oily, then glycolic and salicylic acid might actually be more beneficial for you.

Serums

Never really heard of before the 2000s, serums have become some of the most popular products on beauty shelves today. But what are serums, and why have they become such staples in our skincare regimes?

The word serum comes from the Latin word for whey, as in the protein-rich liquid that is extracted from milk during pasteurisation. In bodily terms, serum is the part of blood that contains all the dissolved nutrients, not including the blood cells. When it comes to skincare, serums can be thought of in this way: products that contain high levels of active ingredients in a concentrated form. They are usually meant to be used sparingly and for a particular purpose, be it anti-ageing, reduction of age-related pigmentation changes, or reduction of skin oiliness.

Usually, serums are designed to be used after cleansing and before the moisturiser/SPF step in your skincare routine. The idea is that the highly packed nutrients and active ingredients will penetrate into the skin and reach the deeper layers without interruption by any of the protective barriers that are created by moisturisers and SPFs.

Serums tend not to be in the form of creams or balms; instead they are clearish gels or fluids, or oils, depending on the ingredients they contain. There is generally much more focus on active ingredients, such as antioxidant-rich vitamins A and C and AHAs, in serums than in other skincare products.

Sunscreens

If you only use one product in your skincare regime, please let it be an SPF. As you're hopefully aware, ultraviolet (UV) light is the number one cause of skin damage and ageing, not to mention skin cancers. Reducing exposure to UV, as you would with any form of radiation, is absolutely key to good skin health. In recent years, UV filters have become more and more sophisticated.

However, they have also come under scrutiny, with some claiming that they can have damaging effects on both ourselves and the environment. A lot of this is sensationalist journalism rather than actual science, and indeed, even the main culprit identified as "toxic" in a famous *New York Times* write-up, oxybenzone, has not actually been shown to cause any harm to humans.

I would therefore say: be sensible. What we do know for sure is that skin cancers can be lethal and that UV is the main cause of them, so we would be particularly silly to not use UV filters in our skincare based on some overhyped and underresearched hearsay. At least until we have further solid evidence to the contrary.

What does UV light actually do to the skin?

UV is high-energy light that is constantly emitted by the sun. Life on earth would not be possible without it, but it does have its drawbacks as far as our skin is concerned. Its high-energy particles hit the various structures in our cells (DNA, collage, elastin, etc) and cause irreversible damage. This in turn sets in motion a whole cascade of inflammatory reactions, which cause further harm in an attempt to control the incoming threat.

Over time, repeated UV exposure can cause permanent changes in the cells, including overproduction of pigment by damaged melanocytes and interference with normal cell division. Eventually this may result in skin cancers.

UVA vs UVB

You may have heard of two types of UV light, UVA and UVB. What is the difference, and why does it matter when it comes to choosing a sunscreen?

These acronyms actually relate to two different bands of UV light, with UVA accounting for over 95% of the rays reaching our skin, and UVB accounting for the remaining 5%. While UVB light is higher in the summertime and penetrates less deeply into the skin, it tends to cause more irritation and inflammation than UVA.

What is meant by SPF?

SPF or sun protection factor is a number relating to how much UVB a sunscreen ingredient filters out. It does not relate to UVA. For example:

- **SPF 15** – blocks 93% of UVB rays

- **SPF 30** – blocks 97% of UVB rays

- **SPF 50** – blocks 98% of UVB rays

So really the difference is not huge. This being said, when it comes to UV radiation, every little helps. What an SPF number doesn't tell you is what it does with the UVA light.

For UVA, only certain ingredients are effective screens.

To protect yourself from it, you need to make sure the label on your sunscreen says it is "broad spectrum", meaning it covers a broad spectrum of wavelengths, i.e. all the UVA wavelengths of light. In the EU, this has been formalised in the star rating system, which goes from one to five stars, depending on the effectiveness of the UVA screen. In products designed for use in the EU, the symbol UVA in a circle means that the UVA protection offered by a product is at least one-third of the SPF factor (i.e. an SPF 50 will essentially offer at least an SPF of 10 against UVA). It's all a little confusing, I know.

What about chemical vs physical screens?

The great debate in the world of SPF factors usually centres around what is better, a chemical sunscreen or a physical screen. You can tell which is which from the ingredients list on the back of your product.

Chemical sunscreens are essentially "organic" (meaning that they contain carbon-based compounds) that absorb UV and cause it to dissipate in the skin. The UV they absorb changes the chemical structure of the compound and stops it penetrating deeper. These include compounds such as avobenzone, octinoxate and oxybenzone, as well as many, many others. The concern around this type of sunscreen is that the chemicals that are produced when these compounds are changed by the UV light they absorb, might in turn cause damage to the skin (by heating or chemical changes) and the body in general.

Physical (or "inorganic") sunscreens are basically salts of metals, such as zinc oxide and titanium dioxide. Unlike chemical screens, physical sunscreens reflect and scatter UV light away from the skin surface to stop it penetrating any deeper and causing damage.

Which is better?

That is a difficult question. So many people have tried to answer this and I have to admit: I don't have the answer. It is really down to personal preference.

Personally, I prefer chemical screens. They are lighter in weight, tend to be less comedogenic (meaning that they are less likely to block pores and cause breakouts) and you don't need to use as much. Physical screens need to be applied quite thickly to achieve the level of protection they say they provide. In fact, you may need to apply as much as two teaspoons to the face and neck alone to obtain the cover stated. Similarly, they may produce a reflective white film on the skin, which might be problematic for darker skin types.

In February 2020, the European Commission reclassified a popular physical sunscreen, titanium dioxide, as a category 2 carcinogen. Albeit this was from inhalation, but it has cast some doubt over its relevance as a sunscreen.

Chemical screens, by contrast, don't need to be applied as thickly and don't have the issue with white films. They can be incorporated into moisturisers more easily and they can have better textures. However, they can cause skin irritation in some people.

How often should I apply sunscreens?

Sunscreens do wear off through the day, particularly if you are swimming or sweating (even if they say they are water-proof!). With physical screens, I'd say once every two hours is a good guide; with chemical screens maybe not quite so often.

Usually I recommend applying suncreen 30 minutes before going out in the sun, and reapplying after swimming.

Do I need to wear sunscreen year round?

Yes. As I mentioned, UVA is present year round and is one of the major causes of skin cancer, so constant protection is necessary.

Specific skincare for particular issues

Dry skin: moisturisers and humectants

When the world-famous dermatologist Zein Obagi said in 2018: "When you use moisturiser every day, you run the risk of making your skin older, not younger," people who had been using it religiously for years were rightly taken aback. But there is certainly something that rings true in his logic – most of the moisture in the skin comes from within, and by using a moisturiser you may interfere with its natural hydration levels by drawing water towards the surface, away from the supporting dermis layer.

The jury is still out, but personally I think that a bit

of additional moisture is what some people's skin needs. Moreover, modern moisturisers aren't only about hydration – they can do so much more.

Their primary job *is* obviously to hydrate the skin, reducing tightness and improving suppleness. This will usually be done by humectant molecules such as glycerin and hyaluronic acid, which are long-chain sugar molecules. The way they work is by drawing water molecules to themselves and holding onto them. You also want to look for fatty acids in a moisturiser, as these can help maintain and support the normal function of the skin barrier. These molecules are known as ceramides – you might see them labelled as ceramide followed by some letters on the ingredient list of your moisturiser.

For those of you with dry skin (particularly if you suffer from conditions such as eczema) and lower levels of sebum production, moisturisers can be very effective preventing cracking and tightness.

Retinoids for oily skin and acne

Retinoids are essentially a group of chemicals related to vitamin A. Vitamin A itself (retinoic acid) is a fat-soluble vitamin that is key to many processes in the body, including supporting the immune system and maintaining eye and skin health. Vitamin A also ensures the proper function of your heart, lungs and kidneys. As a group, the retinoids have strong antioxidant effects and can influence a whole host of other functions at a microscopic level. The way vitamin A works is by passing into your cells and binding to your DNA, affecting gene expression and causing all sorts of changes within the cells as a result.

In the skin, retinoids are a particularly important category of ingredient, in both anti-ageing products and active skincare for oiliness and acne. They come in various forms, the most widely known being retinol, the alcohol form of vitamin A.

There are a number of major benefits to using a retinoid on the skin. They are clinically known to:

- Accelerate skin cell turnover

- Reduce pigment production

- Limit cellular and DNA damage

- Reduce pore size

- Unclog pores

- Reduce sebum production in acne

- Exfoliate

- Stimulate collagen formation in dermis and thus reduce fine lines and wrinkles

- Reduce dark circles under the eyes

There are various groups or "generations" of retinoids, which have been developed by pharmacists over the years.

These groups vary in their strength, side-effects and uses. I always suggest that, if you are starting on a retinoid for anti-ageing, you start weak and build up gradually. This is particularly the case if you have sensitive and reactive skin, or skin that is prone to dryness or cracking, as retinoids can unintentionally exacerbate these issues. A good way to start is by trying an over-the-counter retinoid such as retinal palmitate, retinaldehyde or a low-strength retinol and then gradually increase the strength over a period of a few months. For severe cases of acne, a prescription retinoid, such as tretinoin (a topical cream) or even isotretinoin or Roaccutane (oral drugs) may be needed.

8

MAKING CHANGES FROM WITHIN:
LIFESTYLE, DIET AND SUPPLEMENTS

Topical skincare only goes so far into the skin. With almost every skin condition, whether it be an inflammatory disorder (such as acne) or an autoimmune disease (such as psoriasis), the cause is more likely to be something coming from inside than the skin surface.

The same goes for skin ageing. Although UV exposure from the sun accounts for a lot of the changes we see over time (it's by far the most important external cause of skin ageing), poor gut health, bad nutrition, smoking and stress are also major players in the process of skin degeneration, regardless of one's genetics.

This is because, when it comes to the deeper layers of the skin (i.e. the dermis and below), proportionally most of its nutrition comes through the blood supply. Therefore, diet and general health are probably the most important factors in optimising skin health. Like topical skincare, though, any change to your diet and lifestyle (including taking supplements) needs to be consistent, and to be given time to bed in. You need to persist with a new regime for at least a few months to notice any changes.

Diet and lifestyle

Lifestyle plays a big part in skin health and your first step should always be to address the things that are obviously bad for you. When it comes to diet, there are many guides out there about how to eat properly for your skin (and general anti-ageing), but the key factors are:

- Maximise intake of antioxidant-rich fruits and vegetables.

- Try to stick to a largely plant-based diet.

- Reduce intake of animal-based products such as dairy and meat (when we eat animal flesh, bacteria in the gut release a molecule known as TMAO that has inflammatory effects throughout the body).

- Avoid excessive intake of sugars and processed foods.

- Cut down on food preparation techniques using "dry

heat" such as frying, roasting or grilling, in favour of "cleaner" heating methods, such as steaming or boiling. Dry heating methods increase the formation of advanced glycation end products (AGEs) in the foods, which are molecules that stick to structures in our bodies (e.g. collagen) and stimulate inflammation, ultimately reducing our collagen levels (not to mention causing other serious effects in the body!).

Where do supplements fit in?

Supplements, in my opinion, are an easy way to ensure you're getting the optimal levels of all the vitamins and micronutrients your skin needs to function to its fullest. It's not that they are a substitute for living and eating healthily; more that they should be used in conjunction with a healthy lifestyle. More and more studies are showing that dietary supplements in particular can have good long-term effects on the skin, utilising the blood supply as a means to deliver the important building blocks it needs to maintain the structure of the dermis and even reduce pigmentation and other effects of UV damage.

For how long do I need to take supplements to really see a difference?

Taking supplements isn't a quick fix. Most supplements will take at least a few months to produce any noticeable changes, and benefits are only evident with consistent use. This is obviously dependent on the individual supplement and its active ingredients; indeed, certain supplements (for example, adaptogens) shouldn't be taken for more than a month at a time without a break.

What sort of things should I look for when choosing a skin supplement?

As I mentioned, there are certain things we can look for in supplements that can help boost the skin from inside over and above diet, particularly if your diet is less than perfect. Broadly speaking, these fall into the categories of micro-nutrients, macronutrients, pro- and prebiotics and super-foods. Superfoods is a bit of a muddy term as it is pretty hard to define but I like to think of them as ingredients from nature that have exceptionally high nutrient density. Many nutrition experts are suspicious of the term so I use it lightly and just as a way of categorising.

Micronutrients

These are small (micro) molecules that act as building blocks and cofactors (substances that assist with biological chemical reactions) in many body processes. They include:

- *Vitamin C (ascorbic acid)* – aside from its strong antioxidant effects, oral vitamin C has been shown to increase production of dermal collagen and elastin, have photoprotective effects against UV light, particularly when taken with vitamin E, and can help reduce hyperpigmentation in the skin.

- **Vitamin E** – this fat-soluble vitamin works together with vitamin C to increase its effectiveness.

- **Vitamin A** – fat-soluble vitamin A has numerous effects on the skin, both topically and orally. It can be taken in two forms orally: via retinyl esters (e.g. retinyl palmitate) and via provitamin A carotenoids, such as beta-carotene. The retinyl esters have more beneficial retinoid-type effects in the skin than the carotenoids. They can help treat acne and other skin conditions, particularly in severe cases.

- **Vitamin D** – also fat soluble, vitamin D has important roles in wound healing and normal skin function. It is normally made by the skin in response to UV light exposure from the raw material cholesterol. Sometimes vitamin D deficiencies can occur in people with darker skin living in colder climates where light levels are lower, so supplementation is necessary.

- **Trace metals** – trace metals are important cofactors in many processes and enzymes in skin cells, including collagen manufacture and melanin (pigment) production. They are also important in maintaining the health of the hair and nails. This group includes metals such as: copper, zinc, selenium and iron.

- **Amino acids** – these are the building blocks of collagen and elastin, as well as other structural components of the skin and skin cells, and a wide range of them are necessary for the normal structure and function of the skin. Collagen, the major structural protein in the skin, is mostly made from three types of amino acid: glycine, proline, hydroxyproline and alanine. Some supplements contain all three but taking a complete protein supplement such as hemp protein or soy protein will ensure you're getting enough of them.

Macronutrients

These are bigger (macro) molecules. There are three main groups: carbohydrates, fats and proteins. All three are essential parts of any healthy diet and important in different ways for good skin health.

- *Proteins* – collagen is not only one of the most abundant proteins in our bodies, but also one of the most important for our skin. I've mentioned above (in the section on amino acids) the building blocks we should look for to provide our bodies with what they need to make it. Make sure you get plenty of vitamin C, as it's a key cofactor in this process.

- *Carbohydrates* – long-chain carbohydrates, such as glycerin and hyaluronic acid, are essential in maintaining hydration, suppleness and the structure of the dermis. Since these long-chain carbohydrates are essentially chains of sugar molecules (which we get in our diet), taking a specific supplement for this purpose is not necessary.

- **Fats** – a variety of fats are important in maintaining the normal structure and function of the skin, for example sebum (oil) production, and vitamin D synthesis. When it comes to supplements, two of the most beneficial for your skin are omega-3 fatty acids (also known as alpha-linoleic acid) and omega-6 fatty acids (linoleic acid). Both of these are considered essential fatty acids, meaning they can't be made by the body and therefore need to be ingested. They can help improve hydration of the skin, and reduce lines and wrinkles. Omega-3s can be found in fish oils as well as various plant sources, particularly flax, chia and hemp seeds. Omega-6s are found in walnuts, pumpkin seeds, sunflower seeds and oil, and soya.

Collagen drinks – do they actually work?

Drinks containing fragments of collagen, usually from either bovine (cow) or marine (fish) sources, have become popular in recent years, but there has been much debate over whether there is any point taking them if you already have a good protein intake in your diet. Collagen molecules are extremely bulky, and cannot be absorbed without breakdown in the gut. As a result, most collagen drinks contain a blend of collagen fragments (peptides) and a variety of collagen-stimulating micronutrients (such as high-dose vitamin C). Collagen is made in the body from a number of different amino acids (the tiny building blocks of proteins), which come from dietary proteins. In my opinion, most of the benefits of these drinks come from the additives, which are doing most of the work to help the skin build its own collagen, rather than from their collagen content. Indeed, most of the studies regarding collagen drinks tend to be fundamentally flawed in their approach and are more often than not commissioned and paid for by the manufacturers themselves. Having a good protein intake in your diet and a supplement with plenty of antioxidants, including vitamin C, will do just as good a job.

Pro- and prebiotics: gut health and the gut–skin axis

The impact of gut health on the skin is becoming increasingly apparent. Research has highlighted the importance of the gut commensals (i.e. the normal array of bacteria, yeasts and other flora living on the surface of our gut wall), not just for the health of our immune and other body systems, but also in the development of many skin disorders (including acne, rosacea, eczema and even psoriasis) when they are disrupted.

Certain conditions can upset the levels of "good" bacteria in our gut, leading to colonisation by opportunistic "bad" bacteria, which can cause inflammatory changes in the gut barrier, as well as problems with absorption and other more systemic widespread effects. Since all the organ systems of the body are intricately related, an imbalance here can have major effects elsewhere.

What can we do to ensure we have the "right" bacteria living in our gut?

The answer to this is multifold. Firstly, eat a healthy diet rich in fruits and vegetables. It is believed that animal products such as meat and dairy may have damaging effects on normal gut function, so I'd try to stick to a plant-based diet as much as possible. They are not only better for the environment but also have the effect of optimising gut transit time by virtue of the higher fibre and antioxidant content. Bacteria in the gut really like to feed on complex plant carbohydrates, which allow them to produce their own antioxidants, which can in turn play a role in reducing stress on the gut and maintaining its protective barrier (similar to the skin's).

If gut transit time is too slow (for example in diets low in fibre), not only is the exposure time to potentially damaging toxins and free radicals increased, but the bacteria also run out of their preferred carbohydrate sources of fuel, and start to consume the protective mucus layer of the gut and break down animal protein as an energy source. The breakdown products of certain animal proteins contain molecules such as trimethylamine N-oxide (TMAO), which has inflammatory effects on the gut and the rest of the body when it is absorbed. This isn't good for the gut, or the skin, or any other body system.

Conversely, excessively fast transit time isn't good either. It's a balancing act. In situations where there is an imbalance of bacteria or inflammation in the gut, often the transit time is markedly reduced, resulting in reduced absorption of key nutrients and in some cases diarrhoea. Inflammation can cause the "good" bacteria and yeast to decrease and other opportunistic bacteria (such as strains of *E. Coli*) to colonise the gut and make the situation a whole lot worse. Antibiotics are a huge problem in this regard. They obviously have a desired effect when it comes to treating an infection, but a major drawback is that the bacteria in the gut are often sensitive to them, too, so they should never be prescribed unless there is a very clear need for them.

An ideal gut transit time is 24–48 hours. This can be aided by a good, balanced, largely plant-based diet, and by optimising the type of bacteria in the gut. There are a two things we can do to help this; first, try and incorporate more prebiotic and probiotic foods in your diet, and secondly, and perhaps more efficiently, take prebiotic and probiotic supplements.

Prebiotics

This is the name given to the types of food that the gut commensals like to use as fuel sources. By consuming these over time, we can improve the type and abundance of "good" bacteria and yeast in our gut. These are generally plant-based sources of oligosaccharides (i.e. long-chain complex carbohydrates) and include things like:

- Artichoke
- Chicory root
- Kefir
- Olives
- Potato starch
- Radicchio
- Asparagus
- Garlic
- Kombucha
- Pickled/fermented vegetables
- Wheat bran

Probiotics

Probiotics, meanwhile, actually contain the microorganisms that are thought to have beneficial effects on health, i.e. bacteria. The two best-known strains found in supplements and probiotic-rich foods are:

- Lactobacilli
- Bifidobacterium

Probiotics are often found in foods that have been fermented (similar to prebiotics), and there is often a crossover between the two groups. Supplements containing mixed strains of probiotic bacteria have become popular and there are many on the market. Always choose encapsulated forms of supplements, as sometimes bacteria are killed by the stomach acids as they pass through, significantly reducing the effects. Encapsulated forms tend to reduce the risk of destruction in the stomach and many suppository forms (i.e. up the bum!) are available as an alternative. For daily intake, I'd suggest looking for a supplement with around 30 billion colony-forming units (CFUs)

Probiotic-rich foods include:

- Apple cider vinegar
- Kefir
- Kombucha
- Sauerkraut
- Cultured vegetables
- Kimchi
- Miso
- Yoghurt (both dairy and plant alternatives)

Superfoods

As I say, I use this term lightly. It just helps to group together a number of different ingredients that have diverse and widespread health benefits. They are as applicable to the skin as any other body organ. In any case, superfoods are taken by most to mean nutrient-dense natural whole foods, which tend to have high antioxidant and anti-inflammatory benefits. The list is seemingly endless but includes foods such as:

- Acai
- Almonds
- Baobab
- Blueberries
- Chlorella
- Flaxseeds
- Grapes (particularly red grapes)
- Hemp & hemp seeds
- Kefir
- Matcha green tea
- Parsley
- Pumpkin seeds
- Seaweed
- Spirulina
- Sunflower seeds
- Yucca root
- Alfalfa
- Avocado
- Basil
- Chia seeds
- Curcumin/turmeric
- Garlic
- Grapeseed
- Goji berries
- Kale
- Maca
- Mushrooms
- Pomegranate
- Rosemary
- Spinach
- Sumac
- Thyme
- Walnuts

Sleep

Sleep is super-important for skin health, and can be enhanced with a number of supplements, too.

How does sleep, or a lack of it, affect our skin? Firstly, circadian rhythm is important for hormone levels, which in turn can influence the skin's physiology. Secondly, the functioning of the skin changes from day to night, and good sleep is a requirement for this to proceed as normal.

The problem is that it's often hard to come by, particularly in this century. Good sleep hygiene techniques such as avoiding blue-light screens close to bedtime, taking time to relax and unwind and a hot bath might help a little but sometimes we need more. Fortunately, there are many supplements available to help stimulate natural sleep, without using prescription medications. These include chamomile, lavender oil, magnesium, melatonin (not available over the counter in the UK), passionflower extract, tryptophan/l-tryptophan (5-HTP), valerian root. As with other supplements, a blend of a few of these ingredients can often really improve effectiveness.

Conclusion

You could argue that how we appear to age today is more a collaboration than a foregone conclusion. The considerable increase in our understanding of how our bodies mature is changing the way we age both inside and out. Diet, exercise, skincare and treatments have advanced significantly over the last 20–30 years, meaning that it's possible to feel and look much better than we might have done at the same age 50 or so years ago. With people living longer, retirement ages being pushed back further and the stresses that are placed on our bodies becoming more medically recognised than ever, knowing how to look after yourself (and why) is essential.

Plastic surgery and the new world of aesthetic medicine sometimes gets a bit of a bad rap, with high-profile enthusiasts taking things a bit too far. Indeed, before she died, Joan Rivers famously remarked that, "Betty White's bowels move more than my face". But this perception of Botox, and indeed of the beauty industry as a whole, is (hopefully) changing as we learn to use these treatments in a more nuanced and intelligent way. We tend not to recognise when things are done well, only when they're overdone.

And, as I hope I've made clear, important, too, is a

holistic approach to ageing. The whole process of getting older is intricate and complex, and so a multifaceted approach is best – which is why I've covered everything from skincare to fillers. Look after yourselves, all!

Acknowledgements

A big thank you to all the men and women who have helped me look vaguely presentable over the years. I would love to thank everyone individually, but the list would be so long that the book would have had to double in size. Thank you, too, to my husband, Simon, for patiently letting me hog both the bathroom mirror and our study for most of the lockdown.

Much gratitude to Alex Bilmes at *Esquire*, the team at Mr Porter, and Nicola Jeal and Kate Reardon at *The Times* for letting me bang on about clothes, or try out various aesthetic treatments and grooming regimes, for the pages of their publications. Some of those stories or experiences have worked their way into this book. In fact, the idea for this book was Ms Jeal's. She's very good at pushing me into the water.

Finally, this obviously wouldn't have happened without the support and wisdom of Rebecca Nicolson, Aurea Carpenter and the lovely team at Short Books.

Jeremy Langmead

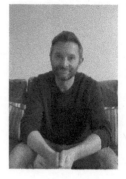

A former editor of *Esquire*, *Wallpaper* and the *Sunday Times* Style magazine, Jeremy was also one of the award-winning founders of the global men's e-tailer, Mr Porter.

He now writes a weekly men's style column for *The Times* Saturday magazine, a grooming column for *The Times* LUXX magazine and contributes regularly to *Esquire* and Mr Porter. He has two sons and lives between the Lake District and London.

Dr David Jack

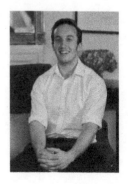

Dr David Jack runs a renowned Harley Street aesthetic clinic which specialises in aesthetic medicine and anti-ageing treatments. In 2017, David launched his own vegan skincare brand.